Aspies Hate Christmas

Amanda J Harrington

Copyright page

To Dale,

Without whom neither I, nor this book, would have turned out quite as we were intended.

Contents

Introduction

It's not all about Christmas!

I chose the idea of Christmas for this book as many families on the spectrum are affected by strong, complex emotional reactions around special occasions.

Whether the special occasions roll around each year, or are one-offs, people with Aspergers and their loved ones, have to cope with the social interactions and challenges these times bring.

There are no simple fixes to how special occasions and social pressures affect people on the spectrum. Expectations often over-rule personal choices when family and wider responsibilities collide with what an aspie would rather do.

In this book, I devote a whole section to Christmas, as this involves particular challenges to aspie routine and personal autonomy. The 'Being Social' section focuses on other social gatherings, from big weddings to parties. Both sections delve into the nightmarish nature of some (most) social events, and the loss of power which leads to us being there in the first place.

Even sociable aspies find it overwhelming to be in the middle of an event packed with people and sensory challenges. This is compounded if other people feel like danger. A great deal of this book highlights the aspie reaction to danger, explaining what can feel dangerous and why.

Anxiety gets a bi mention. It won't be a surprise to anyone how much anxiety – and the behaviours resulting from it – impact on a life with Aspergers. I think it's important to see anxiety clearly, to understand how different it is from worry or nervousness.

In the same vein, I have explored empathy and Aspergers. We can be accused of not having empathy: this might be true, or the opposite of our truth. As people, I reserve the right for us to be different from one another, and to feel empathy or not. Being a good person is not dependent on feeling empathy.

I have also mentioned school and work – two simple words which present complex social and emotional challenges. These are also the areas in life where expectations are daily and on-going. We are expected to go to school, expected to get a job and work. Daily life revolves around a standardised set of responsibilities.

I refer to expectations a great deal in this book. I feel it is vital for friends, family and best beloveds to understand why and how an aspie reacts to 'normal' everyday routine experiences in such a dramatic way. I also want loved ones to understand why a dramatic reaction is not the only response. Just because your aspie leaves the house and goes to school or work, does not mean they feel safe, or are safe.

This book is written from my own viewpoint, as an adult woman on the spectrum. I move the points of view between people on and off the spectrum. Some of the chapters are adapted from my popular blog, Crazy Girl in an Aspie World and are included because people have found them relevant and helpful.

I use comparisons, metaphors and analogies a lot in my writing. I love to find new images to explain the how and why of a spectrum life. Sometimes these analogies are like reading through a dream: this is significant as life often feels like a dream, and I am moving through it.

Not all aspies feel the same way about all social expectations and events. This book is not intended to tell you everything – only people can do that, and then they can only tell you about themselves. Take this book as a starting point to understanding the full stop at the door, the plea not to leave the car, the absence of an aspie when you are all ready to go.

Move on from this book with a new understanding of what makes each other tick, and what can be done to bring happiness and contentment to your lives.

Be good to each other, and remember you can say Yes as well as No.

A word about language

Over recent years, questions have been raised about using the words 'Aspergers' and 'Aspie'. Negative associations with Aspergers have meant some people in the autistic community will no longer use the term and want it to be removed from general descriptions.

I thought long and hard before writing this new book. What language to use?

As an aspie of a certain age, I am comfortable with the words I use to describe myself. I don't want to upset people, I also don't want to alienate those who still use terms that have become familiar, either for themselves or their loved ones.

I consulted people on the spectrum, parents, best beloveds, children. I discussed, considered, thrashed it out mentally and emotionally. And realised that whatever I do, I will not be able to please everyone.

At this juncture, I decided to use words I still value, personally, and which are most familiar to my readers and potential audience. If in future times, they fall out of use, there will be a big re-write!

For now, throughout this book, and in my earlier books (A Guide to Your Aspie and How to Talk to Your Aspie), I use the words Aspergers, aspie and talk about life on the spectrum.

I apologise to anyone confounded or upset by my language choices. No hurt is intended.

Personal choice is vital, and this includes being able to use words which, in my view, have been appropriated by the autistic community. A comparison might be using the word 'hoover' in place of vacuum. We might know Mr Hoover invented early vacuum cleaners, but hoovering is now a verb in its own right.

I'm sure I could have chosen a better example! However, my point is the same. Aspergers as a descriptive noun is separate to the man who contributed to a modern understanding of the autistic spectrum.

The spectrum and the people on it should be our focus. Not as a sliding rule of high-functioning or otherwise – this too, is under debate as a limiting description. Rather, a spectrum full of colour, light, shade, bright, rich, matt, sepia: a prism where we are each our own spectrum, and not limited to one part of it.

1: Being social

The soft light of the quiet day

An empty room, a quiet house, an understanding there is nothing to be done today, or tomorrow: Nothing can stretch out over as many days and weeks as I want.

The loveliness of being home, the joy of not having to be anywhere else. This is what freedom feels like.

There is no loneliness, only solitude. No knock at the door or grasping, grabbing world coming up the street. Clock ticks, hands turn, light moves across the mirror.

Best would be a day of rain, gentle rain that takes all day to finish falling. The outside sheened through the glass and, if I look close, trees blurred within it. Window open enough to hear the rain without letting it in and brief patters as drops blow against the sill.

This is the sort of day that I want to last forever: the peace I think of as I sit in traffic jams or wait for a student to do their work. Surrounded by the lives of others, I yearn for my own, as if it also belonged to someone else.

We all know, in the real world, there is a price to pay for

staying in, not meeting the world, not being the person who can. In those quiet times when the perfect life is momentarily remembered, homesickness washes over me for my own room, falling rain, the soft light of the quiet day.

A lesson in a crowded room

How did it come to this? One small, ill-considered 'yes' lead to being trapped in a room full of people, my instincts screaming at me to run, with nowhere to turn.

How does it happen? Why does it *keep* happening?

I take a breath and cast my mind back to when I arrived, still with a chance of escape, walking unendingly, inexorably towards the door to this room and *going through*. Replaying the moment of entry makes me feel less trapped somehow, as if I am reminding myself that beginnings beget endings and sooner or later I will leave.

Right now, I'm still here, trapped. Surrounded by leering faces full of shining eyes, raucous laughter showing their teeth, spilling into the air, smacking at my ears. Faces turning to me, expecting me to be like them.

Monsters hidden within life, faces unknowable as people I recognise. A terror-filled moment as I wonder if someday I will become like them, without realising I have changed. No physical alteration, a fundamental shift of the beat as I laugh back.

Another breath, and another. It takes a few breaths to avoid breathing too quickly, making myself heady with nerves, quelling what feels like a natural fear but on the outside is me being awkward again.

How many - it comes to me - how many - between breaths - how many - times have I been stuck here in this room, this changing, gameshow-screen room? Always the same room, full of faces, sounds, smells, reaching hands: as if the rest of life were a dream and this clenching nightmare the only true reality.

No, sometimes there are not enough breaths to hide my oddness or to make this acceptable. Standing up, I mutter what could be an excuse and push my way to the door. On the way, I accidentally kick up against someone's chair and am forced to hesitate, to grimace-smile an apology.

They smile back up at me, not seeing my face, my eyes, the fear: not able to connect in the intangible way that lets them see I am on the verge of tears or screaming, my chest stopped with danger.

Outside I wait in a quiet place, hoping no one will come

to look for me; also hoping someone might come and make it all better in that magical way that has not happened in adult life.

Standing sideways to hold the wall, breathing, looking down at my feet, head resting on the cold, comforting bricks, one hand raised to support me as I try not to give in to my ragged nerves.

Time passes and if I do not leave for good, or cannot leave, I return to the room.

I look at my hand lifting to the door, letting my fingers touch lightly on the wood, feeling the surface for a remembrance of the cool, embracing wall. Promise myself this is a temporary event and I will be leaving.

The Toilet Sanctuary

It's a temporary safe place, a sanctuary beloved of aspies everywhere. Special occasion meltdown looms, people distort into their monstrous, gleaming forms, the door to the outside is blocked by relatives and expectations. What else can you do but run to the loo?

It's acceptable, you see, to use the bathroom. People think nothing of you walking along the corridor and vanishing into the facilities. It would be a different matter if they saw you hurtling out the exit followed by your devils. You know how worked up they get about *that*.

Going to the toilets is a fantastic stand-by for times when you want to scream or smack someone. It's unfortunate you can't stay there the whole time.

Toilets are great. Generally clean-ish, they involve a quiet space with a seat to sit on and are within the main building so free wi-fi can be accessed. They are usually in a warm room too and, guess what's best?

Have you guessed?

It's the **locked door**. They have a locked door! And you are the one locking it!

Even though you are expected to re-join the main awfulness any minute, in theory you can stay here all night, and no one could make you come out.

That is my favourite part, you know, when I first enter the sanctum and lock the door. I sit down and take a moment to stare at the door, and the lock on the door: they are my friends. It now doesn't matter who wanders into the toilets, they will not be coming in here.

That whole business outside, the one with people and the feeling that I need to be not-myself, that is gone. My only friend, not counting my phone, is the locked door.

The joy of those minutes as I check my pages and go on Facebook! The fascination of news stories I read to delay returning. The temptation to update my status with some acerbic comment - and then realise I can't because there are people out there on my friends list (irony!).

If it's a bearable event, I eventually leave the toilets and sigh my way back to the group. Only the closest or most intrusive of companions will ask why you took so long; most people wouldn't dream of drawing attention to it.

If it's a bad event, or a bad reaction to a good event, the toilet can be hard to leave. I have shed tears in there and then realised I need to spend even longer so I don't look like I've been crying. I've even pretended to be physically sick to explain my blotched, tear-stained face.

And more than once I've emerged from the sanctuary with the knowledge that, this time, the temporary reprieve was not enough and I Must Leave - only to be told we can't leave yet, it would look bad, it's a nice event, we have to stay until at least x o' clock, you'll have a good time if you give it a chance.

It will do you good to socialise for a change!

Here in body, I stand amongst the crowd, physically present and as sociable as I am going to get, my inner mind focused on escape.

As you get older and less inclined to entertain the nonsense of expectations, you see less of toilets and more of exits. Even then, there is something nostalgic about the quiet place, the sound of a party muffled by tiled walls and your quiet self protected by high walls and a locked door.

Thank you, toilets everywhere.

It'll be fine once you get there

We all have to do things we don't like.

I don't want to go either, but you don't hear me complaining!

It was fine last time.

You always make this fuss and then it's fun.

Why do you have to be so difficult?

I haven't got time for this!

Just put your coat on.

There's nothing wrong with you.

Everyone is expecting you.

You'll upset your aunt/uncle/grandad/cousin/stranger

How unsociable/uncaring can you be?

It won't hurt you.

It'll all be over before you know it.

You have no choice!

If your (insert less able relative/friend/acquaintance) can do it, then so can you.

You went last time.

I'm not arguing with you anymore.

You are so mean.

If you don't go, you'll never get used to it.

If you don't go there, you'll never go anywhere.

How many times do we have to go through this?

Why do you make such a fuss?

You can do it if you really try.

It isn't that hard!

You're just being silly.

I don't know what goes on in that head of yours.

It's only because I care.

You're going, and that's that.

If I don't make you, who will?

You enjoyed it last time.

Not again!

Just grow up.

don't

make

me

go

It'll be fine once you get there.

Don't make me go

Come on now, be honest, how much of the previous chapter looks familiar?

If you were the one trying to persuade your aspie to go somewhere, you might think you wouldn't use words or phrases like those. Are you sure?

If your aspie read the list, how familiar would it look to them? Or perhaps you recognise the words, but feel they are justified because your loved needs to do what's good for them?

Maybe you use gentle encouragement? Kind words?

How does it look when you get upset because they want to stay at home? Do you think your aspie knew you were upset because you were going to miss a special event? Or had to go alone?

In your mind, you were (quite rightly) upset to miss out on going or trying to enjoy it by yourself. You have a right to be upset when you miss out on something good.

To your aspie, you are upset because of them, **they have upset you**, they are making you sad. It is logical – they wouldn't go, you wanted them to go, you were upset because of them. And that is true too.

You might be feeling some hurt towards your aspie. They feel **mean** for not going, your face says they are mean. This is in the heat of the moment, the reaction. But next time this happens you both remember how upsetting it was and both, in different ways, replay it as a bad event.

I have been this aspie so many times, as well as the aspie who goes out and is determined never again to go - *never*. Being determined never to go again doesn't stop me feeling mean for saying no.

I realise I'm being difficult, I just don't want to go.

I'm sorry you're upset, I didn't want to go.

I don't want to be mean, but I'm not going.

I know I'm mean for not going.

I'm sorry I am mean.

How about a perennial favourite – you're just being **silly**. Maybe you wouldn't mean to put it like that. You know Aspergers itself isn't silly, you know the anxieties and behaviours associated with it aren't silly.

It is possible that at some stage you might have said, 'This is silly, let's just go!' Perhaps you didn't call your loved one silly, you used the word to describe a situation where they felt unable to go somewhere with you because of a bundle of terrible feelings which made them too insecure or unhappy to leave the house.

There are plenty of people who have called us silly over the years. Teachers are great for this, or extended family who arrive in time to see the carnival end of you trying to fit a rhombus aspie into a square life.

The word 'silly' is often used with children, so when it is used for older children, teens, then adults, it feels especially spiteful. It is a demeaning word because it dismisses the reasons and emotions behind a person's behaviour, making them out to be a spoilt, bratty child who is difficult instead of well-behaved.

It is an all-encompassing word designed to minimise a

disability to the extent that we are putting it on and need to grow up and out of it - get over yourself and stop being silly. Can you think of a better way to make someone on the spectrum feel silenced?

And speaking of minimising, what about 'It isn't **hard**'? This is well worn too, a favourite used when a social event involves family. It isn't hard to meet family, they are your people, kith and kin: you all belong together.

You're safe with family, why would it be hard to meet them? You know them well too, so again, easy. What could be hard about walking into a room full of people you know? (My stomach clutched for the moment it took me to type it).

Actually, it's very hard sometimes. I know that sounds a bit *silly* and I'm probably making it *hard* for myself and being *mean*.

It can be hard to overcome the sense that the only safe place you have is where you are right now. Fear is a strong emotion and a strong motivator. At this moment in time, your aspie is strongly motivated to not go and do the thing you want to do because they are afraid. It might not be hard for you to go and do it; that doesn't mean it isn't hard for someone else.

Walking into a room full of strangers can be easier than moving through a room of people you know. Strangers tend to be curious for the seconds it takes you to come in and then they fade off to whatever they were doing before.

Family, though: they see you, recognise you, want to speak, get you over, come to you, claw at you, grab, cajole, squeak in your ear, drag you to meet someone you're supposed to know, wonder if you are married, still live at home, working at last.

There is no escape with family; they even know you well enough to follow you to the toilet or call over the locked door to see if it is you in there. (It is always you in there).

They assume they know you better than anyone else, even if you spent your entire childhood feeling like the odd one out. And because they assume they know you, they make more assumptions about how to treat you.

It boils down to family deciding that every member of the

family is more or less the same. If they feel happy and relaxed, all are happy and relaxed; if they are pleased to see a big group of relatives, then we all are.

Why would you be worried? It makes no sense to be worried about being with your family! And if it makes no sense, it doesn't exist.

It'll be fine once you get there. This phrase is likely to be used by someone who thinks you were fine last time because nothing terrible happened. You didn't go up in a puff of smoke when you attended the event. Maybe you sat quietly on the end of a sofa and wished for death: importantly, you kept this fact to yourself, meaning it was fine once you got there.

Regardless of you explaining how you felt at the time, while begging to leave, or talking about it afterwards – to the person determined on sociability, it was fine when you got there. Their memory, naturally adept at pointing out proof of your survival during and after the social event, has a blank spot when it comes to what you said and felt about it.

Your strained, staring face, phone clasped to your chest

like a talisman? Inconsequential. You were a little shy at first, but fine once you got there.

Fa-la-la and off we go, the merry-go-round of lies moves to a dark undercurrent of music. Once you are on it, you are fine.

Similarly, keeping company with pets/children, hiding in the toilets, admiring cars you can't see in a dark car park and discovering an aspie-sized space at the back of the bushes, is all fine too. No one noticed your efforts to avoid adult human contact, you were fine once you got there. Simply being there means it was fine.

Seriously, do not say this! It was *not* fine, it was survived. Bruises don't have to be made with blood.

Cousin Gerald can do it. Yes, bring out the relative who manages despite being worse than you. If cousin Gerald can do it, you certainly can! Look how he manages, and he enjoys himself, bless him. You don't catch Gerald complaining and hiding in his room.

Comparisons are most useful with inanimate objects – with people, not so much. The custard cream doesn't melt in the tea, why do you? The jam sandwich can hold itself together, why can't you? Oh look, that wonderful chocolate biscuit has oats! Why don't you have oats?

Comparisons are familiar, and the implied criticism is never far away. Gerald can do it: he doesn't hide, avoid, do whatever it is you do. Good on Gerald, I'm pleased for him. But we are none of us the same as other people – there will be things I can do that Gerald cannot.

And how unfair to Gerald to hold him up like this, as a paragon, when all he is doing is living his life. Most Geralds would be appalled to find they were used as a stick to poke someone else, especially if the Gerald has faced their own difficulties and overcome. Don't use comparisons, and don't use poor Gerald either.

If you don't go, you'll never get used to it. This is an easy one, and a short one too. For the benefit of anyone reading, aspie or otherwise: **You never get used to it.**

You get better at hiding how you feel. And you might get better at choosing social events you might enjoy. But you really don't get used to it, not if it isn't what suits you or makes you feel happy. We're back on the merry-go-round of lies, and I'm sick of that music.

I do understand the point of view of friends and family who want their loved one to come along and be happy. I get it, honestly, I do. I know sometimes it feels like we are being deliberately difficult, especially if you repeat the same performance every single time – frustrating is not a strong enough word! I can imagine how this feels.

It's frustrating from our end too. Deeply, deeply annoying and exasperating. Good grief, if we could change, we probably would.

(I say probably, but, that merry-go-round…)

((Weddings, really? I wouldn't change if it meant going to weddings))

We did mean it when we agreed to come, and for almost a whole day afterwards. We know you are trying to hold your temper, squeezing words out from between gritted teeth.

It's just that there are relative amounts of suffering: the suffering we feel when you suffer, and the suffering of going out to do the thing you want. Your suffering is horrible, but the suffering of going out?

No, please, that suffering goes on and on, it lasts forever and an evening. Your suffering is truly awful, but we know what to expect with it. Terrible as it is we will stick with what we know.

And when it comes to '**If I don't make you, who will?**' That's why we love you and hate you. We love that you try, that you care and hope enough to keep trying to get us there. It's true, despite everything, we love you for trying.

We hate you for it too. In the end, being made to do something that might be good for us feels like pain.

I don't know what goes on in that head of yours. I don't know what goes on in my head either and sometimes there is nothing in there but fear and confusion.

You have no choice, the biggest lie of all (can you hear the music?). You know what's true? There is always a choice, even if it is the wrong one. We all have choices and one of the ways we make life better is to choose what we do and what we don't do.

One of the most important messages you can give someone is to let them know they have choices – another would be that you support those choices. Don't worry if it seems unconventional – Aspergers is not ordinary, you know.

Once we are allowed to make our own decisions, or we discover we can make them whether allowed or not, the weight of responsibility is lifted by the sense that it is okay to do what seems right for us. Having choices makes a person feel free and secure at the same time.

Anxiety fades because choices are not claustrophobic, they don't box you into one route with no room for self-preservation. They get you off the merry-go-round. Choices mean you can say No and Yes.

It's okay to say No.

This one isn't on the list but should be. It really is okay to say No. It's also okay to say Yes. Leave us to choose and see what happens, you might be surprised.

(Honestly, you might. Eventually, you will be surprised, and sometimes they will be happy surprises).

It's okay to say Yes.

The Forced Social

Parties are *fun*! People are *fun*! Being social is *fun*! Fun, fun, fun.

Being on your own is sad, lonely, okay for a change but we all need people.

Positive or negative perceptions, based on what society judges acceptable, normal. Exceptions are recognised, but in general, being with other people is fun, being on your own is not.

Being sociable is enjoying the process of other people, of not forcing it or learning how to do it. Turning up to be with others does not mean this will happen naturally. Granted, it seems to happen naturally for other people – send them into a party, they smile and dive right in. Drinks after work? Apparently great, not horrific at all.

The number of times someone has said to me, 'You'll enjoy it once you're there!'. This assumes an automatic process: being with other people is fun, therefore, once you are with other people you will have fun. Voila!

And once there? I used to linger, waiting for it to be fun, or waiting for it to be over. Now I linger by the door because it holds the promise of escape and I know it will let me leave, which is more than can be said for the person who brought me here.

I linger by the food too, as eating food is something you do at parties and it doesn't look out of place. It means I can avoid talking to people by taking a long time over food: the time-filling aspect of finding plates and glasses, precious seconds deliberating over what to eat, desperate extra time looking for a space to eat.

There is only so much time a person can spend eating, standing by the door and hiding in the toilet. Chatter and social stuff are in every locatable space. Floor to ceiling people, enjoying this elusive fun you have been promised

Simply being in the room feels like socialising against my will, guided by a well-meaning host – and they do mean well, most hosts actually want you to enjoy yourself. They don't realise they are part of the problem.

If I am lucky, I spot a dark corner with one of my own kind lurking there and a spare chair. This is the holy grail of a forced social gathering.

I totter over, maintaining careful no eye contact so that the other person knows I am not coming to be sociable. I drop *slowly* into the chair near them, covertly shifting my chair a few inches further away from them as I land. They give me a grateful side-glance which lands somewhere in the air near my nose, pleased I moved the chair to avoid being uncomfortably close.

Silence, then. The silence of a deep corner, punctuated only by me surreptitiously, methodically, secretly shoving at nearby chairs with my foot in case anyone gets bright ideas about joining us. The silence of shared suffering is a rare thing and treasured.

'What time is it?' I might ask the room in general, glancing to the ceiling. My new soul-mate will know exactly what time it is and why I am asking.

'Half an hour to go,' they reply to the curtain.

I can't help but sigh. Silence falls again and we both bask in it, in the safety of a shared dilemma.

At some point our host will sally over and ask, brightly, if we are having a good time, their gaze passing between us to imply they have noticed us Being Sociable.

We both liven in the same manner, faces animated momentarily, hands shifting, body language agreeable and happy – or an approximation of the above, as observed in other people.

'Yes, thank you!' We say and the person leaves, content they have made me happy and I am enjoying the party.

'Quarter of an hour,' my new companion murmurs to the room, and their phone emerges from where it hid when our host arrived. I bring mine back out too and, securely hacked into our host's neighbour's wi-fi, we spend 15 happy minutes in mutual solidarity.

Later, in the empty reaches of the night when I am safe at home, the phone will light briefly with a friend request and I discover what my soul-mate is called and what their real life is all about. The conversation impossible at a party is easy online and I have found a new friend.

Being Social is really about finding people who have a clear view of you and meeting them in the right places.

Why I won't sit next to Gladys

Did you know that when we were kids Gladys made my life a living hell? I've told you this before, why don't you remember? No, I'm not exaggerating!

Being kids is no excuse. Neither is *just* being kids, or young, or any of the lies grown-ups tell themselves to pretend it doesn't matter when one small child bullies another.

When we were 'just kids', Gladys and I, we played together because we were about the same age, even though Gladys was more streetwise than me and played rough games.

She told me stuff I didn't understand, and she could outfight her brothers. I was supposed to be friends with her because we were related.

How was I supposed to be friends with someone who laughed at me whenever I said anything because I talked funny and made no sense? Being alone with Gladys was a short, sharp lesson in other people and what they might really think of me.

Here we are, years after your abject betrayal of littler me and you *still* expect me to get along with Gladys?

I don't care whose birthday it is, I don't care whose wedding it is, I don't care what occasion it is or which social nicety means I must share a table with her: I will not sit next to Gladys.

I couldn't care less how she's changed – that is a tacit admission she needed to change! I have met her in the years between then and now and she does not have me fooled.

At the occasion, I know Gladys will be dressed up and made up with a hat set on styled hair; she'll be wearing a shiny outfit that makes me want to cut out a piece and keep it. But as I arrive, she will sideways smirk at me, the up-and-down eye flick at what I am wearing.

The difference is, these years later I know Gladys is a cruel fool and that we were never going to be friends. I know she laughs at me to cover the fact she doesn't know what I'm talking about. I realise that Gladys might even be nervous of me.

In any event, the biggest problem I ever had with Gladys was being made to spend time with her when I wasn't old or wise enough to look after myself. I may not always feel wise now, but I can stay away from Gladys.

Your event can either go on without me or go on with me sitting in another place. I will not sit next to Gladys. Sit me with strangers instead - maybe those work colleagues bundled together on the same table. Or old Bert, who is no relation but gets invited to everything and drinks to himself in the corner.

Yes, I'll sit with Bert and watch him bend towards the table, held up by his drinking arm. I might even talk to him a bit, while he melds into the table. In the distance, I can keep an eye on Gladys and her brood and wonder how genetics really work.

Later, when the time is right, I may begin to enjoy myself. Or I might decamp to the toilets. Either way, I will be confident I asserted myself and that next time, no matter what, there will be no suggestion of sitting next to Gladys.

And maybe, if I'm very lucky, I'll find out why Bert does get invited to everything and exactly who he is.

The safe list

Everyone has a list of people they get along with. It isn't an exclusive list, entry to my life is not dependent on having your name on the list. But each person who has made it, is there for a reason.

I speak of lists because aspies operate with one hand on the tremor of the universe and the other hand holding a list. While emotions storm, swirl, move in eddies physically incomprehensible, our heads are trying to make sense of it by deconstructing life into a manageable set of facts.

If I have the facts, then I know what to do. Breaking down scary situations into facts makes it possible to understand them. Understanding is the key to the universe, or at least that's how this aspie operates.

This relates to people as much as anything else. Some people will always make the safe list, some veer on and off it like a toddler in a plastic tractor and some creep onto it, slowly, carefully, after years of getting to know me. (They deserve a medal once there, really).

Then there are the ones I never expect to move onto my

safe list because they make me feel unsafe. They fit alongside strangers. All strangers are on the unsafe list until confirmed as proper people who mean no harm. This is acceptable thinking – stranger danger – it's not safe to trust everyone we meet.

Families don't expect us to have strangers on our safe list, they do often expect us to accept people who don't make us feel safe.

People who have sullied their record badly, are familiar, related, life-long cast members in our personal dramas. They are expected to be on our safe list just because that's how it is. They have not earned a place, they have not made us want to forgive or trust them, they have not (in our eyes) done anything to warrant changing our minds about them.

Time after time, I have been judged for not wanting some people near me.

Accused of being unreasonable and childish, I might discuss or defend my position, explain again why this person is not my person. It rarely does any good.

I am not sure why people in families think it is acceptable to tell an aspie to grow up in the same conversation as ignoring their judgement. Don't grown-ups make their own decisions? If I make a decision, why should someone else's views win out over it?

Why should my decision, backed up by facts and logic which I can quote to you, be denied oxygen, yet a mushy-feelings decision, 'because family', be the one I should accept? It's amazing how seldom people in family circles are willing to listen to an alternative viewpoint about someone they know.

We are all people, separate individuals happenstanced by thousands of years of random, genetic encounters. Is it not logical to think that amongst this vast backdrop of contributors, there will be personalities that do not get along?

This logic gets me nowhere. What place does a theoretical, abstract argument have in a loving family environment? We are not talking about science, we are talking about people – the same people who applaud you for knowledge as a 12-year old and accuse you of thinking too much once you hit 20.

The family logic extends as far as: Why would a grown person (me) hold a grudge against someone (Gladys) just because of how things were years ago? Even if things happened when we were children, don't I understand that people change? Don't I know that this person, as they are now, is wholly different from how they were then?

This aspie begs to differ. Children change their behaviour, people develop as they age. Does this change their intrinsic nature? Perhaps, I know it can happen. Does it mean they are automatically safe because they seem to have changed? Can I be the judge of that, please?

When I look across the table at the unsafe person nearby, I see them as they were then, face twisted in ugly fury, eyes glinting at their own power. When they laugh at a joke, I know which part they find funny because it is a joke making fun of someone. When they ask a friendly question, I answer and hope my eyes don't give away my appraisal of them.

I end up trying not to look at this changed miracle of a person. Looking at them brings back the times before and the way I feel now. I still see it, no matter how they behave, how expensive their clothes, how reliable their behaviour.

In turn, they see me as the weird, quiet kid, as awkward today as I ever was. In their new sensibility, perhaps they pity me? Or maybe they think none of that and are as unknown to me as I am to them.

There is an impasse with people who don't feel safe. In all honesty, I don't ever want them on my safe list but by admitting as much, by trying to explain why they make me uncomfortable, I am a critical person who misunderstands someone genuine.

The other person can think what they like about me: by being able to act normally when we meet, they show themselves to have moved on. As I don't manage this, I am grumpy and irrational, and I need to grow up.

Years pass, people change, I find the will to be there in the same room without reverting to the small child. I made it through many trials before returning to this one; I am somewhat proud to realise who I am and what I do, and do not, like.

Here, in this place, at this event, I need to sit near my old nemesis who will never be on the safe list and I am expected to like them and show that I do.

Sometimes, one more trial is not what I need. The first step to making trials easier is in accepting I have real feelings about this person, feelings which are not silly or imaginary.

This time, why not sit us a little further apart? Out of direct eye contact, near someone I don't know well anymore, or haven't seen for years. If it is to be a family event, will it shake the earth to have me next to ones whose faces light up when they see me, all grown and new?

I guess it brings me back to good old Uncle Bert and his way of being a safe place. I don't understand how some people who I don't know well, and who might not be on my list, feel safe when others don't.

Perhaps there is something in this illogical sensory life after all. Or maybe the tremor of the universe is not meant to be understood, only felt.

2: Christmas

A very aspie Christmas

'Come in! Come in! and know me better, man!' said the Ghost of Christmas Present.

And there, summarised by the spirit who wishes to enliven and embolden the hearts of all mankind we have three good reasons to hide from Christmas: I do not want to come in, I do not want *you* to come in and I do not want to know you better.

Maybe at another time of year I could be emboldened or enlivened. At Christmas, my comings and goings are likely to be from one safe place to another, with hard diversions into unavoidable human contact. The thought of welcoming in the rest of mankind is frankly unacceptable.

I do love Christmas. At least, I love the lights and the decorations and the cold, dark outside with the warm gold inside. I love the bleakness of the weather, drab scenery filled with shadows, glowing shops empty of people, late-night streets, sparkle lights prickling the darkness.

All that human stuff, with people even more social than other times, it galls me.

At Christmas we love each other, and our hearts warm for traditions we don't manage the rest of the year. Shops madden into activity and people you will never see again are compelled by the power of Christmas to wish you well.

We climb up onto the idea of Christmas, carried abreast as if it were a giant, tinsel-tossed ship taking us to glitter-sand isles of goodwill.

How is this fundamental change, this voyage of Christmas spirit meant to take place? I have plenty changes in spirit all year round, often in the same day: as yet none of my spirits has thrown me into a fervour of sociability.

If I am confused by a Christmas splendour of softened-hearts, then other people are perplexed by my apparent indifference to them. I have no need to be drawn into anyone's heart, be it figuratively or (saints preserve us) physically. If you draw me in, stop it.

I have never made a secret of my love of solitude so why is it surprising that I don't change my feelings for Christmas? Solitude is not an old coat, hung in the cupboard til after New Year. I don't have a gold lamé jacket in there, waiting to be pulled on with my smile.

Keep your hugs, your mistletoe, your bottle of good cheer, which I can't drink anyway. Keep your best cake and hand-made mince pies (I lie, give me those). Keep your expectations that I will be one of you for the season.

I am not one of you, no more than I was in November or will be again in February. I am one of me instead and quite happy with it.

I am not Bah Humbug, honestly. I do love Christmas and am happy if you love it too. Allow me to be like the spirits as they take Ebenezer round the snow-filled streets of his childhood - let me also tread unseen and unheard as others take their warm welcomings.

To me, windows glowing in a dark street are far more welcoming than a door opening to beckon me inside.

Ho-ho-ho?

Or humbug?

Decorations, or an empty room?

Tales of joy, or what we do on a weekend?

All-hail-fellows-well-met?

Swigging alcohol? Or put the kettle on?

Beautiful presents under a darling tree? Or just the corner?

Lights sparkling in the edges of the room, twinkling outside in the garden, gather, wind-blown over the old willow. Or a garden lit by streetlight?

Does it have to be a choice?

In families who would otherwise celebrate Christmas, it is a choice they might be forced to make to help loved ones cope with the changes of Christmas, the sharp sting on non-routine. It becomes the choice between doing what is best for your family, and doing what is expected.

Some families shun part or all of Christmas to make it bearable at home; others lean on their reluctant aspie, explain to them, ease them through the season.

If Christmas is a must, children can only be roped in for so long. There is no explaining to teenagers who are now old enough to know their own mind. They've heard all the excuses for making changes they don't like, and they're not doing it anymore.

Older still, and here we are as adults. Some of us at home, some of us living away, alone or not. Christmas rolls around and, for goodness sake - still? After all these years of me telling you how much I dread it? Still?

The reasons and excuses why Christmas must follow a usual path reappear, as much a reminder of the season as the dust-covered, broken box full of tinsel.

I used to think that adulthood meant independence, freedom to make my own decisions. How naïve of me. As adults we are still expected to take part; worse, to be one of the reasoners who play the game, because that's what we do at Christmas.

At the time of life when personal autonomy means Christmas can be ignored, that's the stage when guilt and emotional manipulation are at their finest. Now, as an adult, I am expected to understand why we need to do things I hate. No! I don't understand! I did actually think the whole point of being a grown-up was to make my own life!

Sorry, exclamations galore. I get worked up about how much of adult life is steered by what other people want. Not everyone's adult life, but a fair few of us.

I wonder how many of you reading this are a guider, a reasoner? Someone who is adept at steering their aspie to do what must be done? Come on, it's fine to admit it, I can't hear you from over here.

Sometimes it's a good thing to be able to reason your aspie into action. I recognise that my desire to be at home is not always what's best for me, that it has long-term consequences which lead to me not going anywhere and my life diminishing.

What I would like you to think about is, how long does an aspie who *hates* Christmas (insert dreads, fears, despises, etc) have to put up with the charade? When does the rule book support this adult over the other adults? When does the fellowship and goodwill to all men apply to the member of your family who dreads the season?

When does it apply to the aspie who fears visitors at the door? Or noise and music? Or by mid-December is leaving the room because you didn't fast-forward the Christmas advert in time?

When does it apply? When they move away? Or are they expected to come back on repeat because it's Christmas?

After all, being an adult is different, isn't it? Now we don't fear something like Christmas, that's childish. There's nothing to dread, that's silly. And hate? Too strong a word. Now you are an adult, you know that hate is best avoided, used sparingly like pepper.

Christmas dawns and each of us is meant to embrace our inner child and celebrate the season. The aspie takes their inner child by the hand, wanting to where there are no visitors, or requests to do this one more thing. We can only hide for so long.

When you call your aspie down into the main room again, probably with visitors imminent or already there, they are not alone. Their inner child comes too, a younger self who watched, aware that fun was to be had and couldn't work out why.

They stand, wide-eyed at the door, ready for flight, and while you are stifling the thought, 'No, please, not again,' they aren't thinking anything, but seeing –

- the roll-out of Christmases gone by, visiting everyone before, and then the day when everything is to be perfect and not a harsh word or raised voice. Lights lit, food eaten, presents unwrapped with keen eyes and camera handy -

 - smiles, everywhere, eyes and smiles.

- room full, bright, loud, space on the floor alongside a present or next to Aunty's knees as she sits on the sofa.

Today a space for them, as an adult, where Aunty used

to sit. A space to fill with gladness and appreciation for what we have, are given, love, take, consume, desire, rip out once a year and in the name of Christmas.

Trembling at the door, knowing you think, 'No, please, not again,' seeing it on a reel, this Christmas rolling into the others.

One year, one of these years, it becomes too much to sit in a spare and empty seat while others smile.

The Christmas Aspie

The perfect image of Christmas, what would it be? Joy and colour, light and noise? People happy? Full homes?

Where did my solitude go? The safe places? The get-out clause (no pun intended) if it's all too much? If I vacate, have I Failed at Christmas? How dramatically awful!

At Christmas, we are meant to be brighter, better versions of ourselves with more kindness and time to spare for our fellows. With this level of pressure, is it any wonder aspies don't cope?

I don't want to fail at Christmas, I just want a Christmas that suits me, rather than shaping my Christmas to fit everyone else.

I don't do parties, or most gatherings. I rarely send cards. I don't want to go on a mad round of visiting and having visitors. I wish strangers a Merry Christmas if they do it first or say it to a shop assistant who looks fed up.

Christmas tends to bring out the hugs in people, the kisses (why do people do this?) and the pushing to have a drink, when I don't drink.

I appreciate the idea of Christmas as a time of giving, of becoming a little of the person I hope to be, without caving to the pressure of doing what is expected. There is a vast difference there.

I like fairy-lights, tinsel, the tree, window decorations, spray snow, real snow - the glittery side of the season. I like to dress the cat and take his picture for Facebook and take the dog out in his Santa sweater.

I like the old fire at Christmas, the light in a darkened room, the sense that this season brings us closer to all the people who went before, sitting in their safe places while the wind howled tales of dread and demons.

I love the lights on trees as I pass by, bringing magic to winter nights, reminding me of childhood days when I went fairy hunting in summer and laid traps for elves in winter (sorry, yes, I was that child).

Most of all, I like the quiet days after Christmas when everyone has gone home, and I am safe to sit by my fire, dreaming away time as winter slumbers on.

What do you expect of your Christmas aspie?

I expect myself to look forward to Christmas each year, to hang my magical lights, to live in my snow-coloured imagination, to admire the shine.

I don't expect others to advocate Christmas, to stick lights on spiky trees in pouring rain, to listen to Christmas music or cry when Judy Garland sings.

My lack of expectations, my calculated lack of them, takes account of others being themselves and me being me. This is brushed aside each Christmas.

At this time of year more than any other, old issues come out to haunt me: do Christmas this expected way, it's what is right.

For the rest of the year, people somewhat remember my limitations, depending on the situation. In other words, they remember I am an aspie. Come Christmas, and Musts, Shoulds and sneaky little Could-Yous wriggle out of the woodwork.

It's as if my spectrum life switches on and off like a Christmas jumper, swapping one blink of me for another, in honour of the season.

Relatives and friends suddenly *must* visit. Previously, on Life with an Aspie, it was deemed acceptable to see them away from the safe place, somewhere we could impose a time-limit.

Now, they must come to our house or we must go to theirs. And we all must have a Good Time and be jolly and...sociable.

The only thing that saves me on Christmas visits is if people have children. We can talk about Santa, watch cartoons, do some colouring, make bad decorations, and discuss out how the sleigh works and whether reindeer prefer to land on a roof or in the garden.

Children are not the same as adults, you see. They don't expect me to be jolly when I haven't been jolly before. They see the twinkle in my eye or the subtle reaction that means I love their new storybook. They know, for certain, I am really watching the cartoon with them.

Adults need the jolly. The twinkle in my eye is not enough, the limits of my excited speech and pleased demeanour disappoint them. Why can I not take part more? Why do I never make enough effort to show people how I feel?

Perhaps because I have nothing to show them? I feel nothing for their present or their story about a Christmas bargain, or how their friends in Australia put up a tree on the beach. I smiled, didn't I? Yes, that was a smile. Yes, that was the best I could do.

By the middle of the visit, the grey, damp feeling has descended, as if my chest and stomach are packed with sodden, dusty stuffing and I am an eyeless doll. I have no reserves left, nothing to show for the Australian beach tree story I hear every year, no work-around for my disinterest in Christmas bargain excitement.

I am empty. And cannot refill until we get out of here, which seems like it might happen in a couple of hours/lifetime.

There is no extra pot of reserve for Christmas. I used part of it leaving the house, I used another part coming out on yesterday's visit. Some of it slipped away when I climbed out of the car and saw them waving there on their front step, brimming with enthusiasm.

I am here, where I was requested to be, and not even hiding in the garden with the dog. This is the best you will get today.

Why do I always have to be rude and critical, especially at Christmas? What will people think of me? What will they say?

On our way home in the rain-covered car I briefly imagine my story appearing next to the Australian Christmas tree. 'And did you know, she couldn't raise a smile, even though it's Christmas? She might as well have stayed at home!'

Sometimes, like stopped disagreeable clocks, we all agree on something.

A Second Christmas?

One of the unrelenting things about Christmas is that it only comes once a year, so if it doesn't go well, or well enough, you must wait another year to make it right.

First, it's debatable whether we should be trying to make it right or glorious, as per made-for-tv-movies on the backburner channels. Christmas should be what you want and maybe sometimes what you get, instead of what you think it should be.

Having said all that, after spending one Christmas in a paroxysm of discomfort and emotional fatigue, I felt particularly cheated. The thought of waiting a full year and hoping that chance might throw me a decent Christmas just seemed too...harsh.

That was when it hit me. I looked at our two little trees - an inspiration when the big one was too unwieldy - and I thought, Why not have two Christmases as well?

Yes, two Christmases, just because.

Imagine, if you will, Christmas without the hype and

expectation. Without feeling the need to buy the right presents or to make the right food at the right time. A Christmas without the pressure to make it perfect.

Imagine instead a Christmas where we spend a tiny amount on each person and decide on a great meal of what we want to eat, minus the expecteds. Lights are still lit on the trees, decorations carry on hanging, Christmas itself is redolent in the air.

So that's where we were. After one traumatic attempt at Christmas Day, we had a few hours before Christmas Number Two. To the rest of the street it was the Monday between Christmas and New Year but to us it was a special day.

We dashed into town with an agreed amount of a few pounds each, buying teeny presents that would be wrapped each by themselves, as if they were going under an elf's tree.

The present buying was *fun*, with the challenge of seeing how much we could get for our money. Aspie son enjoyed his present shopping for possibly the first time in his life - the pressure was off, he knew how much to spend, he knew we were all spending the same amount: it worked so well.

When we opened the tiny presents on our second Christmas morning, we sat around and took it in turns. Great minds had thought alike, and each of us – me, aspie son, eldest and his partner – had all bought as many presents as we could.

It took quite a while to open them all, but there was no worry over the correct reactions, and it was funny! Imaginations brought those few pounds to life. There were comedy presents, hats bought for pennies because Christmas was over, sweets wrapped individually, little ornaments on sale.

I can honestly say it was one of the best Christmases, and definitely up there as a great present-opening event.

It turns out the real magic of Christmas is other people, and how much we can enjoy it without the pressure. Getting presents for others, and receiving them, does become special and happy when the stress is taken off.

I know this might seem obvious to some of you, but this

specialness and happiness was not obvious to me. I knew it was meant to be there, what I was supposed to be experiencing, it just never seemed to work out that way.

I think I felt more joy in those moments than I had since being a child at Christmas. I rediscovered it, and I wasn't willing to let it go.

Each year since then, we have considered a second Christmas. We haven't done it every year, we only do it if the day itself goes wrong, or is stressful, or if we feel like it. The brilliance of a second Christmas is having a choice, and that includes choosing whether to do it at all.

The night before second Christmases, I feel the glow of Christmas Eve all over again. And even if we are doing this one without Santa, I have a feeling he approves.

I wish it could be Christmas every day?

I do wish it could be Christmas every day. Let me keep my decorations and the lights, let me wake up to tinsel wrapped round the bannister rails and baubles tickled along the floor by our little cat.

Let there be songs and films about Christmas goodness and happiness, warmth and home. That's what I want.

And what madness inspires this? The *idea* of Christmas is my safe place, my coming home; it's the big blanket I hide under, made bigger and blanketier. Security in glitter letters along the wall.

It's a symbol, bringing into the real world the feelings I would like to keep with me all year round.

When I watch A Christmas Carol, I identify with both parts of the story - Scrooge in his lonely life, kept separate from other people by his carefully-constructed barriers; then Scrooge as he becomes, warm and merry, with people to love when he lets down the barriers and embraces life.

I've read Dickens' book and it's a much more sombre affair than most of the films. It emphasises the seriousness of Scrooge's separation, leaving us in no doubt that he is a bad person. He has destroyed lives and gone on regardless. He has been a terrible influence in the world, harming himself as much as others.

Does this sound at all familiar to other aspies? If you're honest, how many times have you thought about the harm you caused by your behaviour? By avoiding responsibility or dismissing people's emotions as less valid than your own? Or rushing on, afraid of finding out what you mean in the world, content to be left alone?

In the book, Scrooge is brought to a true, deep understanding of his place in the world and the positive effect he can have on others. He doesn't get there alone: as well as the spirits who come to help him, he has people in his life who are willing to reach out to him, his family and those who would be his friends.

By the end of the story, he learns how to reach back to them, living the remainder of his life in happiness and warmth.

To me, it's this glimpse of contentment at the end of the story which resonates with Christmas. I want that! How often do we feel truly content? How much more familiar is the nagging sensation of incompleteness, inaccuracy? Or worse, the sure knowledge that something is in tatters?

What bliss to be able to reach out and grasp hold of contentment, as if it's a physical prize you can hold, cradling it through life.

All too often, contentment is fleeting, felt usually when alone and following the routine and familiar. A different sort of contentment settles when engrossed in a latest obsession, or an old one that we love to re-visit.

I guess that's part of why Christmas is so important to me, too, because it's also an obsession. Anticipation thrills, excitement flickers with the lights, the fresh pine scent as I walk in the room sparks my imagination.

I have a confession to make. The contentment I crave, I want it always to have a buzz too. I can't cope with pure safety without action. I need that zing, the feeling of being safe now, but later there may be wolf-baiting.

Does it sound contradictory? It isn't, not really. Thrilling contentment comes with a life of your own making: tramping through deep-rooted forests, listening to sounds of danger in the far distance, making an ancient fire at twilight.

A life where you can sledge down a steep hill or run against knife-wind on the edge of a frozen lake.

I want to choose my thrills, live with excitement, like you can at Christmas; to anticipate what will happen next, even if I can't always control it. Life's 'thrills' are often the wrong kind, unseen, unheard until they sweep me up

What I want is my own hand on the reins. If we're going sleighing tonight, I'm in charge of the reindeer. I don't want wild horses clicked on by someone else.

If there's a knock at the door, I want it to be a best beloved. I don't want unwelcome visitors rain and thunder.

I know when I think this that I'm not embracing how people see Christmas or even Scrooge's final lesson. No, I'm not ready to let in the world and treat every person as part of my fellowship. Was Scrooge really ready? Here is a quote from the end of the book:

"Some people laughed to see the alteration in him, but he let them laugh, and little heeded them... he thought it quite as well that they should wrinkle up their eyes in grins, as have the malady in less attractive forms. His own heart laughed: and that was quite enough for him."

Scrooge, portrayed as a chuckling old gent at the end of the films, is a wily goose in the book. He knows not everyone shares his vision or agrees with him, but he doesn't care. He does what he can, he lets his own heart laugh and is content with that.

How boring would old Scrooge be if he only laughed and gave his money away? Far better to have the wise curmudgeon alive within him, truly appreciating life because he recognises what he was before.

That is what we all must do, at Christmas or any time of year: recognise our true nature so we can make changes without losing the special elements of our individuality.

Like Scrooge, we may need shocks to see things clearly,

though I sincerely hope ghostly visitations are not part of this. Examine the past, the present and futures to see not what we *want,* or *hope* will happen, but what will come to be if we don't change our present course.

I am too imperfect an individual to suddenly change into a best version of myself. I *can* change, we all have that capacity, but I cannot become a wholly different person - and nor would I want to be.

Let me too keep the knowledge of what went before, content in my dark forests as well as by the shadowed, fiery hearth.

3: I said, No

It's not my birthday

Un-birthday, non-birthday, just another day - all of them sound better than saying, 'It's my birthday'.

Birthdays are regular, inescapable events that roll round, bringing with them the equally regular and inescapable expectations of other people.

"What are you doing for your birthday?"

"What are you getting for your birthday?"

"Are you treating yourself? We went away to Paris for my birthday and next year I'm getting Jim an experience day on a helicopter."

I know that last one is quite specific, but people do very specific, special things for their birthday, often trying to top what has gone before or create dramatic experiences to celebrate coming, screaming into this world.

For my birthday I am always reminded of the Hobbit approach to birthdays where the birthday person is expected to arrange a big party for everyone and buy presents for all the people in their life. I actually like (LOVE) the idea of giving other people presents instead of receiving them myself but setting the focus on others is what birthdays feel like.

I have to appear to be happy (It's your birthday!)

React suitably to presents (I could love them and still only look vaguely pleased)

React suitably to visitors (open the door)

React extremely suitably to going places specially for an occasion centred around me (deep breaths, deep breaths)

All of the above are reactions arranged around other people but starring me as the central player. This is the nightmare of getting married all over again.

The eyes are on you at birthday time. Whether you try to react suitably or not, the attention is very firmly fixed.

And if you don't like birthdays? Well, apparently this is an alien concept, especially if nothing horrible has happened to make you dread that date on the calendar. Dread of the birthday itself is not an acceptable reason. You're also not allowed to dread visitors or presents, or even singing - how can anyone over 10 enjoy the singing??

This year was different. My eldest son is jollying off to Japan again and will miss my birthday, so he asked if I would like an early birthday.

I considered it: the wrong day, not my birthday, only me and my sons here, a small array of presents opened nearer lunch than breakfast, no visitors, no singing and no going out with a face on.

I grabbed that early birthday! And spent most of it in pyjamas. I reacted well to the presents because, being my sons, the presents were exclusively chocolate and books, so, you know, no forced reactions needed.

I stifled the niggles of nerves first thing in the morning. The negative associations of Birthday were strong enough to creep in even though it was my unbirthday day. Stifled them right down, faced the day, and enjoyed it.

For the record, eldest son started singing Happy Birthday at bedtime, then cackled. Some things are truly inescapable.

And my actual birthday?

In honour of it, perhaps I ate chocolate or read books. Maybe I didn't do anything, my own special non-reaction to the day. To be perfectly honest, I don't remember my actual birthday, nothing to report.

Bliss.

The Paralysis of Fear

Saying and doing the wrong things are familiar and terrifying to me. You would think after a lifetime of No-Tact I might be used to it by now. The irony of being an expert at something which only brings me trouble!

Isn't making the effort to do it right worth some mistakes? Isn't speaking my mind a good thing? Why do I worry so much?

Well, it's the **Fear**.

In some relationships, there comes a point where saying and doing nothing is preferable to doing it wrong. Where I can't stand the freezing, paralysing, stultifying fear of making another mistake. I am terrified of getting it wrong.

You see, fear is not a constant, but is consistent with certain people. If I know someone will react badly to yet more stupid, dumb-ass, thoughtless, tactless mistakes from me, I am more afraid of making mistakes with them.

I can no longer cope with the Look that says, 'You've done it again. *Well done*, you really spoiled it this time!'

How could you forget? You knew how important it was!

You didn't really forget! It was too vital, you're just pretending.

How could you, when we had that enormous row last time and you promised to try harder?

How could you let me down again and again?

How could you hurt me like this?

In the end, I have been labelled as someone who does not, cannot care, because a person who cares *remembers*. And a caring person who forgets has a good and proper reason for forgetting.

Faced with this emotional, accusation-filled outpouring, what can I do but apologise and hide? My other option is a headlong fall into meltdown. Neither of these helps but if I can choose, I'd rather hide than lose more control in a meltdown. Both responses are a kind of hiding: one actual hiding, the other losing myself in a storm.

The next time it happens, I do remember something

important - I remember the fear. That fear is twisted up into my forgetfulness and mistakes. I remember that the other person was angry and upset and I was to blame (or was blamed, which is a different thing but feels the same).

I remember the badness of it, the sense that I wanted the fear and stress to end. I wanted to make it okay again.

I sit and wish it had gone differently – a very familiar feeling. Going over what I forgot, I relive the flash of fear now intrinsically wrapped up with my forgetting, mull over what I could have done to remember and finish with the dull certainty that I will do it all again.

Somehow, I think it is worth promising myself I will never do it again, as if a promise is the magic of remembering.

Looking at it now, I know that what I am resolving never to do again is go through the fear. I promise to do better, but really I am promising to avoid the terror of failure and its heartless consequences.

I may still forget but I now avoid situations where I am relied upon to remember. I still make mistakes but now avoid those people who railed against me for doing so.

I have become a closed book to sections of my life where important people and places live. I move on, and on, holding myself apart from expectations snapping at my heels.

Fear is a motivator like no other. Love and kindness are essential, but fear recalls situations and people in a way no other emotion can. Proximity of fear reminds me of times I have been terrified, letting it into new situations totally removed from the old ones.

Paralysis and avoidance can be positive, if it means you are not trapped, spot-lit in drama, chastising yourself for not getting it right while the other person doubles up by chastising you for getting it wrong.

Whatever brave souls may tell you, fear is not a positive emotion. When you face danger, you run from it and learn from the experience, you do not seek to repeat it and be in danger again. Facing your fear does not make it better.

By realising what there is, and is not, to be afraid of, you free yourself to face aspects of life which should not have danger in them, to understand you are terrified of the tiger mask, not the beast itself.

Understanding *why* you are afraid is what makes it better.

The Inner Meltdown

Logic, kindness, understanding, soft words, hard words, hiding, running, screaming into the fresh air: we all have strategies for avoiding meltdown. But sometimes they're doomed to fail.

A meltdown does not have to be a shout into the wind, a banshee shriek. A meltdown can be an implosion within, buried deep and well beneath a widening of the eyes.

The over-riding factor in any meltdown is the immense depth of feeling, combined with an inability to control it. These feelings can be out of control without needing to move or speak or erupt. Inner worlds collapse behind a hand twitching against the cloth.

This violence within, which might or might not make it without, occurs after our best efforts to dampen it. Meltdowns *can* be satisfying, I admit, but most of us avoid having them because life is complicated enough.

The inner meltdown is almost worse than the one other people can see. In there, the real me is screaming: sometimes there are words I want to let out, bounce them over the room, call them back, bounce them again. Other times, there are no words and I can feel that inside part of me clutching to get out.

I can't let it; sometimes I wouldn't know how to let it. She might be loud enough to deafen me, I still can't let her out. The outside me is likely quiet at this point, harmless in my endeavours, one more person in the world.

I may be counting the seconds til I can leave, trying to take notice in case my betraying, stimming finger rises to its brother and makes the -plick-plick-plick- one finger against another. I hold my wrist, my bag, my coat, the edge of the door; I hold whatever is close and keep myself within the gravity I cannot feel.

I expect my voice to come out sounding strange, unlike the me another person is used to hearing. It comes; to me it does sound like someone else because it is, it's public me who goes on doing whatever she does while the other part claws at self-made walls and my traitorous hand rises again to stim the air.

Act, act, be a normal person, be quiet or talk, and leave quickly. The car is a blessing. Falling into the seat, I throw my bag away as if I'll never need it again and plant both hands on the wheel, the traitor hand with its rising finger allowed to tap like anybody taps, even though the music is silent.

The screaming levels to a roar, I drive away. Some distance down the road I park again and take out my phone. Instantly oblivious to the world outside the car, I dive into the phone, into anything away from here, as if I'm wearing blinkers.

Coming up for air, I breathe a few more gasps of safety and am forced to drive again, to the next part of my everyday life, dreaming of the need to scream even as I park and step out again.

What's so hard about Aspergers?

This isn't a question people often ask. What they ask instead is:

'What's so hard about going to the party?'

'What's so hard about school?'

'What's so hard about work?'

'What's so hard about talking to my friend?'

'What's so hard about talking to me?'

and, the favourite,

'What's so hard about remembering one little thing?'

What's so hard? Is this a good time to give a detailed, enlightening answer? Shall I wave my arms in the air and cry, *'Everything!'*?

Or, as it won't be the first time I've been asked, 'How many times do I have to tell you?!' (Always goes down well, coming from someone as forgetful as I am).

How deeply does the other person understand? Should I cut them some slack? I ask myself this, trying to be logical about it. Have I explained it well enough before? Shall I try again? Are they in a mood? Is it a rhetorical question?

Still, 'How many times do I have to tell you?' is what wants to come out.

Why is it so difficult for other people to remember what I tell them? And know that what I said about school also applies to work, that talking to people can be hard? That I can't help forgetting, it's not on purpose?

And mostly, that it doesn't matter what the challenge is: today it is hard, even if yesterday I could do it.

Our heart-to-hearts before today, the times I explained myself, conversations where I put words together in the right way and they came out in beautiful, perfect sense. Times when I think, *I have brought it to life*, how I feel and someone else knows and they care about me.

Then the inevitable moment when they ask again why something is hard or grow impatient at what cannot be done and it's as if nothing was said between us. My beautiful words, hard-won, careful words, are gone because that was another day and you misplaced it.

What's so hard about Aspergers? Every challenge feels different, even when I know, logically, they are nearly the same. And because it feels different, I'm unsure how to deal with it this time.

I can trip over something that was there yesterday, and will be there tomorrow, but today was when I tripped. I'm annoyed that I tripped, I am so done with tripping! I don't need to be asked why I tripped. Do you think I would hide it from you if I knew the answer?

For all the trips and falls in the world, they are made worse by the person close to you wondering at your ability to be yourself, again and again.

Why did I trip today?

I saw the trip coming, then I looked at the heavens and forgot the earth. I tripped, but I did not fall.

I said, No

Words have power. Clusters of them, like sparrows, less effective, as if they leach power from each other and disperse it into the air – chatter, chatter.

No, a powerful word, is powerless if no one listens. Waiting to be heard ends in doing what you refused to do and being cajoled into thinking it was a good idea.

Saying no many times - *no, no, no, no, no* - a parrot bobbing its head as it calls a word it can repeat, might as well not speak at all.

No amongst its fellow words: *No*, I don't want to; *No*, I don't like it; *No*, you said I didn't have to; *No*, it upsets me, *No*, I explained why.

The headline word is no but coupled with a reason it becomes an excuse, a whine, a nag.

Dismissed as such this *No* hurts most when it is lost. It wasn't simply a refusal, it was a full sentence and a reason, an explanation of why *No* is important and should be heard.

An irony of conversation is that trying to discuss a reason why you don't want to do something leaves space for arguments against your reason and chances to dismiss it. *No, because* is pushed out by *But, yes.*

Then there is *No.*

A refusal to give credit often offends – that old sign on shop counters. Also, a refusal to give a reason for No often offends, as if the word does not belong in a sentence by itself.

No is not a sentence, though. You have been mistaken. No is a declaration of intent, *my* intent not to do, agree, accept, capitulate or otherwise take part in the carnival planned for me.

I said, No.

I know you heard, I don't care if you want a reason – I've tried reasons and here I am, having to say No again, after all these years.

I could repeat myself if you like, but this time not like the parrot bobbing his head. If you prefer repetition let me instead raise my voice and scream **NO! NO! NO!** Is that better? Is that what you wanted?

No, I am not overwrought. Repetition lost its appeal for you once my voice changed.

Perhaps you do prefer silence, after all. That I can do. There is no need to listen to me saying *No*, it is an easy fix.

The absence of me is also silence.

The absence of me means I said, *No*.

4: The Adult Aspie

This is Bob, he has Aspergers

Every year my sister holds a Halloween party. It's a mix of adults and children and I usually go off with the kids and leave the adults to do whatever they do in the kitchen (unexpected laughter, drinks in plastic cups, small pockets of serious conversation?).

I love these parties. I get to dress up without being stared at and eat candy. I also get to go to a party where I don't feel like bolting for the door or holing up in the spare toilet. It's so rare for me to enjoy a party that Halloween has become a time of year I now associate with happy social gatherings - that is, as long as I stay with the kids.

This year, someone new is coming. He's the father of one of the children I already know and usually their mother does the honours, dressed as a gloriously gaudy witch. Their mum can't make it, so dad is coming instead. I asked if he'd be dressing up.

My sister's face changed to an eager expression and she powered through the 'Yes, definitely!' to what she really wanted to tell me.

'Bob is potentially Aspergers,' she said, nodding and smiling at me, as if she had told me Bob would be bringing ten pounds of chocolate with my name on it.

'Oh good,' I said, not really knowing what to say but feeling I was meant to be pleased.

'Yes, there's definitely something there,' she went on, looking thoughtfully at her internal list. 'He's brilliant with computers, very good, but erm, he's not actually done that much with it.'

We can tick off the under-achieving part of Aspergers, then? Thanks sis!

'And he's,' she gave a short laugh and paused. 'He doesn't have great social skills, you know. He can come off as a bit strange around people.'

Resisting the urge to ask her how *I* was around people, I waggled my eyebrows and said,

'Sounds like a candidate then. I'll make sure to switch on my aspie-dar and get back to you.'

She looked pleased and confused at the same time. Perhaps she was expecting me to bring an actual piece of tech or at least a recognised checklist for Bob to complete while he's holed up in the spare toilet.

Feeling the need to explain, I pushed my hand behind my waist and said, 'It's a little switch at the back, I flick it off and on when I need to detect aspies.'

There was cosy laughter at this, of the kind when children tell awful jokes and you have no idea what they're talking about.

'Anyway,' I added, suddenly thinking of something, 'if he's dressed up he might be in character, so I won't be able to test his social skills.'

I imagined Bob as an extrovert wizard, you see, playing the role as we so often do. Or a crazed timber wolf, hungry for blood.

My sister looked at me like I'd gone over the edge, obviously not understanding how being in character could affect his personality.

'Maybe,' she said weakly and changed the subject.

I picked up where I left off, drinking my tea while I watched my sister interact with her friend. They were engrossed, and it was a happy few minutes as I dissected the way they related to each other.

I also thought about poor Bob, relegated to the realm of Aspergers because he's not right, an under-achiever and is great with computers but not people.

Hmm, I thought wryly, I wonder why my step-sister thought of him when I walked in?

When are you going to grow out of it?

People expect you to grow out of Aspergers.

Yes, I know, written down it looks ridiculous. How can you grow out of it? What can you do to grow out of it? Is it like growing out of curls or losing your baby teeth?

Can it be shucked off with my first bra? Can I rip it off with wax? Will it wither and die by itself?

Is it like going bald or putting on a few extra pounds every year – at some stage Aspergers will be shed like youth, hair and a waistline?

It hasn't so far, which leads me to suspect I'm not growing out of it. The opposite is more likely true: I'm finally growing into it.

When you are little, being naughty, loud, challenging, running into the door frame, that's just you being you. You'll grow out of it.

Teenage-you likely calmed down a bit: there is less

excited running or traditional naughtiness. You might be challenging but all teenagers are. You probably still bounce off door frames.

Adulthood beckons - then usually has to beckon again because you didn't notice. Are you doing what you should to grow up and be successful? Have you finally outgrown your funny little ways? Do you still bounce off door frames?

School is over, money must be made, responsibilities wait. Who wouldn't want to be an adult?

Family start to expect more from you. Yes, they know you have Aspergers but...

If you can manage *this*, why not that?

If you can do *this* small step, why not the big one?

Cajoling, they persuade you into the adult world, expecting a light bulb moment where you know what to do. I think, in their minds, Aspergers can be leaned around, stepped over, sat beside, as if it travels with you and not within you.

Not all families are like this but quite a few are, sometimes without realising. Subconsciously, the parent of an aspie child and teen might think that Things Will Get Better as their child ages.

Except, look at it again.

The world is small when we are small and as teens the world opens out, becoming bigger and more complicated than before. Why do you think teenagers are difficult? It's not all hormones; some of it is the bleak realisation that Life is enormous.

To an aspie who felt the bigness of the world in the first day of Nursery, this sense of imminent discovery, the idea that the world just keeps growing, is already there. Through childhood and the teenage years, it's hammered home that we have a lot to learn – including the unwritten rules that others know without learning.

Once an adult, you have more understanding, more sense of the depth and mystery in life, in the people out there. How is a person supposed to feel this every day and not be afraid? How can we push forward if today we cannot move at all?

The trouble with Aspergers is that it gives hope almost every day. New skills learned – tick! new challenges conquered – tick! When they come around again there is a justified expectation that they have (tick!) been thoroughly learned, the challenges vanquished. It doesn't work like that.

Like wind on the meadow, Aspergers buffets over life, fluttering inside us. Could any of us explain the Do days compared to the Do Nots? What is so different?

Is it the direction of the wind, or light in the meadow? Is it that the grass smelled fresh today? Instead of doing a tickable quest, I sat instead, pushing my fingers deep into the grass, looking down to spot my fingers in the green.

Growing out of Aspergers is a hope not often admitted or realised, but very much felt by aspies and their families. When he is older, he'll be able to do it. When she is older, she'll feel differently. When I am older, it will be easier. As if the mere fact of aging were enough to change us as people.

Now I am older, and some things are easier, I can do more, I do feel differently.

I feel that I can be myself and not worry about it; I can worry about other things instead! Now I am older I can see more readily when I might or might not be able to cope. This makes planning easier, because I don't need permission to avoid doing something I know will be difficult for me.

If I have a day when I can't cope with something I find easy on other days, it's okay, I can accept it. I know it's not permanent, that like the wind over the meadow, this will pass, and also return. Being grown up means I can say to myself: today we might not, tomorrow we might.

The downside of this is that I have only myself to chivvy, avoiding activity that I might enjoy or benefit from. Adult me can say NO whenever she pleases, and nobody is the boss of me etc. Therefore, if adult me wants to engage in harmful practices, or not engage at all, adult me can and will.

Just like any adult, I can be my own friend or enemy. The trick to being successful and happy, is in knowing myself thoroughly, recognising the times I can be more than I want to be that day.

I'm now self-employed and vary my work to fit NO times, then take advantage of YES times. This isn't possible for everyone, but I believe it's a good goal to work towards, a productive lifestyle which is flexible enough to 'save' you when you need it.

Aspergers does not get left behind. It hurries along with us, a fierce friend who knows our secrets and revels in them, leading us astray, laughing at our follies and bouncing us off door frames.

Growing out of it would be no fun. What would we do with all these amazing skills we learned? With that ability to suddenly talk to complete strangers about random subjects they never expected or to ask them questions they answer without thinking? Or to leave a conversation we don't like without a backward glance? (Try it, you know you want to).

A life with Aspergers is full of questions, often questions

with no answer. Living without questions might make life less bumpy, but being able to pause, to stop what you are doing and consider a question for which you have no answer is why I would never want to change.

Where would I put these wonderful thoughts and feelings carving a creative ravine through my life, making me a shining, spectacular, dangerous, metaphysical creature who still can't work the key in the front door, or the top step on the stairs?

Why would I want the simple ability to always be able to set foot outside my front door when I can be *paused* in the act of leaving by light hitting the glass, just so?

Why would I ever want to grow out of it?

An aspie at work

Aspie stands at the door, ready to go but mournful in the extreme. The clothes are in place (finally), the hair is brushed through, the face as clean as it's going to be without getting the cloth and washing it yourself. And still, there they are, just like at five years old when they didn't want to go to school.

'I don't want to go to work,' they say, a sad robot on repeat. The shoulders slump and they wait, dejected, for you to throw them out into the cruel world.

'I know you don't,' is all you can say because, after what seems like hours of negotiation, you have reached the point of them leaving for work and you don't want to jeopardise this success by showing weakness.

And even so, after all these years of practice, you let slip the worst comment you could.

'It'll be fine once you get there,' you say, in a cheery voice, opening the door.

The aspie turns, aghast, every eye-widening muscle on

overdrive, mouth open in complete disbelief. Your heart sinks. While your face registers mild regret at the slip, your inner voice is NOOOOOOOOOO!

'It will *not!*' the aspie manages at last, almost spitting in indignation. (Though *not* spitting, as that is vile and your aspie hates people who spit).

'I didn't mean it like that,' you sigh, trying hard not to roll your eyes.

It doesn't matter how you meant it, it's what you *say* that matters.

You may as well have said, 'Perhaps giant lizards will eat you today and then you won't have to go to work,' but stating that it will be fine is tantamount to sending the lizards yourself.

The aspie knows it will *not* be fine when they get there. It will be just as bad as they expect. Even if Bob doesn't chew gum or wipe his hands on his trousers, even if Giselle fixes her contact lenses in the bathroom like a civilised human being, even if the boss does not make that coughing sound when there is no need to cough and nothing is wrong with them - even if these things do not happen, the place will be standing, the work area will be waiting, the overhead lights will be aggressive, the phone will ring, the work will need to be done, the clock will sleep on the wall. And you say it will be fine?!

As you gently manhandle your aspie out of the door, you know that work is not dangerous and that aspies should not sit at home all day doing just what they like. There's a whole world out there to be discovered. The irritations which figure so large in aspie conversation are not important, and you know - you really feel you do know - that it will be fine once they get there.

You start the car, knowing the refusal will happen again once it's time to drop them off but understanding that having the aspie in the car means you are almost guaranteed they are going to work today.

Your aspie knows it too. They sit, head down, hands in their lap so they can see their fingers and watch over them. The world rushes past as you drive and your aspie sees only this small part of it, their closed space until they need to get out.

Dropping them at the kerb, you leave them with a happy smile, knowing they will be fine. Resigned, they walk the rest of the way to work and let the door fall shut behind them.

This is the view from outside, readers. Giant lizards do not come, the clock does not sleep, the boss perhaps needs the aspie to send them a link to persistent coughing (again), the work needs to be done.

The whole world waiting to be discovered is over-rated, work itself is a sorry mix-up whereby we live in a cash-based economy and cannot live without paying for it. Working to live includes a lot of jobs which are not great for people who think lights are aggressive or notice how many times Bob doesn't wash his hands.

Being an aspie is not like being a 5-year-old who doesn't want to go to school. Money must to be made, it isn't perfect to stay at home all day (it so is).

Help your aspie to scale up, scale down: look at other jobs that are marginally better, easier to manage. Look at their skills and see if there is something else they can do to make money.

Maybe it's not about lights or contact lenses. Maybe the hunched demeanour and inherent sadness of work is real, not a temporary barrier that melts once your aspie is out of the door.

Maybe the safe space in the car, with you by their side and their fingers under scrutiny, explains to you what your aspie cannot. If it is impractical for your aspie to say no, it's time to think about what would make them say yes.

Years later, with your aspie in one piece and the workplace far behind, they will remember watching the car drive away and that it was not fine.

Look at it together, not from the 'it'll be fine' perspective, but with a 'what can we do to make it better' plan laid out in the distance between you.

Don't drive away.

The whole world is crazy...not me

A world where people never say what they mean unless they have to, but everyone is expected to know what they mean without being told. Where I must be exasperatingly slow not to know what they mean, what they are talking about, thinking about or doing.

A world of in-jokes I'm never going to get but where my own jokes fall flat or make people laugh - suddenly, loudly, surprised, as if they never realised I was funny.

Where if I find something funny and others don't, I accept it. If they find something funny and I don't laugh, I have no sense of humour.

The kind of world where I'm weird for not wanting to talk about soap operas, holidays, promotions, football or how much we all drank last weekend.

A world where they notice if I leave quietly but expect me to stay and be ignored.

A crazy world where my manners are out-of-place, formal, old-fashioned, and I'm supposed to excuse the rest from having any manners at all. Where one badly-phrased question labels me as rude.

An odd world where I need to fit in enough to not be cast out; where I keep going, one bright-covered foot in front of the other, attempting to take my own path while the world rushes by on the big road both sides of me.

The whole world is *crazy,* and I'm in the middle of it every day, one foot, two foot along my little path.

Stopping sometimes at a bend, or crossroads, pausing to let another like me pass by. And for the moment we trade smiles, familiar glances. Sometimes we talk and relish this exquisite peace, of meeting a like mind, our quiet words blocking out the roar of traffic on either side.

Moving on refreshed, I smile up at the empty sky, down at my patterned feet, one-step, two-step, feeling not so alone.

5: Bad days and glad days

Light

Some days it's easy. I say to myself, Why do I ever think things are difficult? This is fine. If it's fine today, then it can be fine every day.

It's a kind of soft-focus logic where I judge each day to come by the one I'm living *right now*, as if it didn't matter how I was feeling or what was happening around me. Today I manage, therefore tomorrow I will also manage. Or even excel!

Logically, I know other days are not as good, or are better. I'm not a dog, I don't live in a state of ever-present belief in a never-changing universe: there will not always be food in my bowl, we will not always be on the verge of a walk or looking for the lead.

Dogs are hopeful creatures: perhaps today the bin lid will be left off and I can to sort out last night's curry, or they will forget we went for a walk already and we can go again!

The simplicity of this belief, and hopefulness, does resonate with me. Again, I know I am not a dog, people are not dogs. But using dog-logic and optimism explains how I can use today's good day to totally convince myself that this was not a fluke, that by the power of my will alone, I can make my tomorrows good too. The bin lid was left off once, therefore it (might, could, may) *will* be left off again today.

I don't believe I can change reality – if something bad happens, I don't expect to have a good day regardless. In general, this belief is based on the idea that, all things being more or less equal, tomorrow can be the same as today, and on we go from there.

I will make each day as good as my best day, because I say so.

It sounds childish, and it is. It's rooted in the sense of control I felt when setting cars out in the play garage or organising my friends in the Snail Club (don't ask). I organised this good thing today, therefore I can organise more good things tomorrow. Simple optimism spills over into hoping I can change my life by expecting to be able to change it.

Even as I type this, I feel a rush of optimism, the hope

being so strong that simply explaining makes me feel it all over again. I cannot tell you the number of times my misplaced optimism has led me into misadventures!

Ah but, this misplaced optimism has also led to real adventures and discovering aspects of myself that would have stayed in darkness had I not thought, Wow, that's totally a good idea, why don't I do it right now before I've had time to think about it?

A friend once said my life was a series of misadventures, and this is true – probably more true to people with organised lives and a realistic level of optimism. Afterwards, when I am wondering if the paint is washable, then googling how to remove wood paint, I can see that it might have been better to think things through and not rely on optimism to replace reality.

The cat would not have a gold tail, the floor would be clean, I wouldn't have ruined yet another pair of jeans and, the usual outcome, I wouldn't have spent money on something I will never use again.

However, in defence of adventures, I hold up Exhibit A: a feather. (Bear with me).

Imagine a peacock feather, bought in a flurry of excitement about Doing Crafts, and how I would become so good at crafts I could give up everything else and magically make lots of money because of crafts. I buy beautiful peacock feathers and excitedly hold them to the light, admiring the shimmering colours. Then what?

I'd never actually planned which marvellous crafts would use the peacock feather, or how I would learn them. I think I expected a crafty osmosis to happen where I'd gain skills I've never had in my life before and know what to do. That would be great.

The peacock feather is enjoyed and put away, and never used. Other feathers are used as practice; they end up sticking to my jeans and the cat. The practice feathers are put away and never used. Move on to the next day, the next plan, the next perfect misadventure.

The crafts are an example of how a new interest is believed to be a new life, the road forward in remaking myself. The new life awaiting me does not need crafts, or even misadventures. It only needs me to believe that what I have thought of today will prevail tomorrow.

Like the peacock feather, it will be something beautiful and unfamiliar. This new me who knows how to do life: she will go to work every single day and never be bored, stressed or aggravated. She will be organised and know when bills are due. She will never run out of toilet paper or cat food. She is a grand creature, a better version, the one people expect when they ask things of me.

Does she exist? Is my optimism completely misplaced? Can I ever re-invent myself into this glorious creature who floats on dawn's light without touching the night grass?

She does, you know. She's the same one holding up that feather, peering at it, oblivious to the fact she is visible through the window, unaware that in the face she makes she reflects the child who stood at the school window, staring up at rainbow crepe paper stuck on the glass to make a light-catching pattern.

Life has always been about colour, finding it or adding it myself. I may not float over night grass, I rarely see dawn, but if we can't look for colour in what we do, then why look at all?

Optimism is colour. It is the rainbow streaming through

rain-filled heavens on its way to the lake, reflecting a version of itself which is imperfect and shakes as the ripples of the lake move it.

It is visible from afar, inspiring, egocentric and generous at the same time. It brightens dark days and its very nature promises the sun.

Dark

Then there is the yesterday I had.

The sort of day where everything is normal, as it should be. I have what I need, I set off in time for work, I walk there and that's a healthy, good-for-me act. Afterwards, I walk into town.

At some point in the middle of town I realised this was *not* the kind of day where soft-focus logic would help. Who cares what I managed on other days? Who cares how I felt then? Who on earth cares?

It was a long walk out of town, much longer than going in. On the way in, I joked with a lady at the crossing as we dodged over between traffic. On the way out, I crossed the street so I wouldn't have to walk near a stranger who had no interest in me - just being near someone was too much.

Suddenly, somehow, in the middle of a normal morning, my fear-calm scale tipped right over and the little weights scattered across the metaphorical floor. I was alone in town on a busy Saturday morning, surrounded by people who made me feel like I was hurting just because they were there.

I scuttled past market stalls, along pavements I've walked since I *could* walk, hurtled past social smokers outside the bar, down the quiet street that meant halfway home.

There are moments where the very air around me seems to close in and, with almost gentle insistence, suffocate me at the same time as giving life.

Taking stock, I knew I wasn't in danger, that the feeling of fear was generalised - all-encompassing, but general. There was no actual danger, nothing waited for me, nothing prepared a place in a darkened room for me. There was only me, on my way home, alone.

Yes, melodrama, but when you have this feeling of being trapped in open spaces, in peril from indifferent, ordinary people who mean you no harm, when every step home is a stepping stone over deep waters; those days are not melodramatic to you, they are just very hard.

I finally came to my street and saw the tree on the edge of the garden where a grey gate hides. I crossed the road where our old dog always liked us to cross, and missed her all over again, needed her next to me, to put my hand in her curly fur and see her patient face smiling up at me. I hurried the last few yards to my front door and closed it.

By the time I got inside I was twisted out of shape, pliable like soft metal; my sharp edges were still there, it was only their direction had changed.

Safe, I looked at my morning and breathed the open air of home. It had been a triumph all the same. I walked through my fear, saw it clear, took it in, softened under its harsh impulses and made it home.

Much, much later, I went out again to the lake and tested the air. It was still clear, the storm had lifted, and I was able to look at the world again, a little at a time.

Every day is never the same. Managing now is proof you can manage again but *not* proof that you should be able to manage all the time.

When they say, 'take each day as it comes', that is what to do and be glad of it. Someone came up with that phrase from the other side of a bad day and gave it to us.

Take each day as it comes and feel triumph when you manage the melodrama of the quiet street.

Anxiety

Anxiety can be annoying: like a cold, gone in a day, nothing to mention.

Or perhaps a streaming cold, the kind you can't hide: it's messy and you don't go anywhere without tissues. It will be gone in a few days.

It's a flu, you get real sympathy – or you would if you could leave the house, your bed, the fugue you lie in day after day as you wonder if you will ever feel better again. In a week or two it will be gone.

It's a pain, an ache, a muscle pulled in time for a game of tennis. It's a kink in your hair, a tweak in your nose, the way the sun catches your face. It's each small thing and each big thing, it touches every other thing in-between.

It comes with friends, a part of other conditions, and then it is Medical. Your doctor will explain it is medical, often in the same conversation where they explain there is Nothing Physically Wrong. They may be kind or dismissive, but they won't think you are ill. Anxiety is not an illness.

And the days it feels like an illness? This is normal, apparently. The great trick, anxiety causes physical symptoms but they don't mean you are physically ill. They mimic, making you into someone who needs to calm down, instead of someone who physically suffers.

You are the person who says **No** a lot. You fudge your reasons, offer hopeful excuses, leap from the car as it pulls to a stop, scuttle through the front door, take off from the bus stop without catching the bus, leave the shop without buying what you need.

Sitting in the darkness at midnight, watching for the moon and remembering when you were little, and it was all possible; a part of you knows it is still all possible, that you are anxious, but it doesn't define you. There is magic in the world and perhaps you are part of it.

The next day you get up and into real life again, anxiety in front of you, behind you, next to you; between you and the world, magnifying life as it creates a barrier you can't quite cross.

There are meant to be ways of coping with it, realising it is something you can defeat.

There are ways, pick one that works, but don't forget -

The breathless moment when anxiety made you feel real danger is mirrored by the breathless awe when you halt in the middle of a busy world and see this moment filling your day: no Time, no Duty, no way of knowing how long the endless moment will last and understanding -

Anxiety is not just the bad side of life.

It may rule you at times, but the side of you which sees inescapable complexity in the world is also the face which stops and sees the heart of never-come-again.

The shaft of light on her hair through the window, rough edges of painted green-wood rimed with frost, bright yellow spider on a black car in the rainy darkness, a lone crow singing a song for its dead mate lying beneath the tree, glistening, spectral blooms on early morning grass, the sound as the wind dies.

Tiny things which worry you also belong to the beautiful, mysterious, everyday wonder of living.

Be anxious if you must, then live the day around it and with it. Take it as a part of you and see what happens the next time you look closer. Don't always run ahead to escape – don't always look behind to see what comes for you. Don't look for the next step.

Be anxious and know it for what it is: a part of the whole you, as you are a part of the whole world. Your life is full of moments, some of them are anxious, some of them bite. Some of them make you cry. Remember to leave space for ones which do you good or make you wonder.

There is still magic in the world and you are part of it.

Waiting for the turn

Anxiety is living next to a busy road and feeling responsible for every car going past, even though you know they are driven by someone else.

You can't stop listening. In your home, separate from the car, unlikely ever to meet the driver; here you are, paused mid-step, face angled toward the door, trying to walk on, trying not to listen to the noise.

You are inside your house and safe, yet strain to hear the cars as they turn the corner at the end of the road. Senses acutely aware of tyres squealing when a driver sets off too fast or tries to speed round the tricky turn on the next road; more squealing as brakes are applied.

and in your mind's eye

is every turn that can be made

and each danger ahead of it

and every big danger that exists further on

Later, when there is nothing wrong and you cannot sleep, lying with one hand clutching the other, listening for cars going by, one, one, two together...eventually drifting in dreams of roads tumbling into motorways, ditches along country lanes, sharp turns, unreadable signs seen too late.

In the morning, waking to the sound of more traffic, you sit up and look at your hands, determined this day to worry over only what can be seen and felt right in front of you.

Closing the doors and windows to shut out the traffic noise, you consider what you have then build a barricade of soft blankets and down pillows to blot out the grating engines.

Closeted in your muffled rooms you look at your hands and smile. Somewhere out there is traffic but you won't hear it today.

Why panic?

A dark alley might not be safe. If I see movement in there, the shadow of someone hiding, I wouldn't go in. Coming home to find my door ajar with someone moving inside when no one should be home, I'd expect danger or conflict. Visiting a friend with a dog who growls: it has never bitten, but I don't feel safe.

These are unsafe scenarios, where I wouldn't feel safe, and where logic dictates I would not be safe. It wouldn't be unreasonable to avoid them because I am acting on logic as well as emotion. It makes sense to avoid a situation where I could be in danger.

In theory, there is no need to panic. Avoid the alley, call the police, do not visit the dog. Panic erupts in the moment of action - being attacked in the alley, facing a thief, seeing the dog lunge.

Logical decisions save us from panic because panic is the emotion we feel to get us out of an actively-hazardous situation. It is the scream after the thought.

What about a scenario where there is no obvious

danger? Can we still face panic? Sadly, of course we can.

Let's go for a big one, that 500 guests wedding. Let's set it in a posh hotel with a sit-down meal and people serving. The multiples of cutlery shine, plates are set on crisp, clean tablecloths over round tables where everyone is the same distance apart.

The room is big and grand, the lighting is gorgeous – probably the most beautiful thing in the room. There are flowers, ribbons, expensive decorations and a lit walkway through these many tables soon to be filled with people.

Place-names adorn the tables and there are staff on hand to help you find your seat. Everyone is properly dressed for this, it is a formal wedding, and there is admiration and regard for the way the room has been created. This is a wedding of substance.

The guests are in their finery. Shoes bought, tuxedoes hired, dresses chosen months in advance, hair – oh, the hair! Make-up, perfume, jewellery, cologne. Raised, intoxicated laughter, joyous voices filling the air as everyone comes into the room.

It fills and fills, and no one looks familiar, all looking like alternate versions of themselves. Acting that way too, because they have changed to suit the wedding. Children look like dolls, extra decorations for this glorious room.

The room keeps filling and I am here amongst it, dressed in new clothes, smelling like the shop still, the edges unbroken, the zips unfamiliar, the buttons waiting to catch my fingers, my hair not right, my face set in the emotionless safe-zone I keep for crowds.

The filling room has some friendly faces and they speak to me. I open my mouth and move my head as if I speak back: no words come out and it doesn't matter, it is too loud to hear anyway.

The table is an unknown. I am guided to the table and there are people sitting down. I find my name and sit, touching my name, feeling its' familiarity yet fascinated to see it strangely written on high-grade card. I wonder if I can take it home. I see it isn't written after all and make a note of the font.

Some of the people look vaguely familiar but I have no

idea if we are related or not. Others must be strangers, but I never take chances at times like this. I must be friendly to everyone, it's what is expected at weddings; if it turns out I do know them, no one will be offended.

The space between people is quite good. I judge it and imagine how far I can move without having to be too close to the others. I hope I am not sitting next to sociables who like to move their seats closer, who lean across tables, reach over to talk with their new friends.

And then the speeches - ye gods, is there anything that lasts longer? Continents slowly drift as everyone turns and listens. Half the room is now behind me and I turn too, to watch the speeches and be amazed at the jokes and not stare at the lights and – good god is that Jennifer?

I see the way the doors open and close as staff go in and out and I know, soon - not soon enough because a part of my life died while the speeches lived – at some stage I will be fed.

Voices rise again, everyone is jolly, they want to talk, they want to know, they see I am not speaking and help me to join in. I wonder if it shows, if I have some secret sigil on my forehead to say I am not the same. Or is this simply what friendly people do?

I sprint miles inside my head to outrun shrouded panic.

Panic comes in places where there is no easy time to leave, and I am overwhelmed with it. Panic helps me see everything at once, the colours of the room, raucous, beating sounds of life, serving people with food, windows blocking the world outside, the door closed.

Panic settles in, watches from behind my eyes as my mouth dries and I see the escape routes but cannot take them. Food comes, more talking, decisions to make. I have no idea what to say, I feel like refusing everything they offer and cannot refuse anything.

Tongs, plates, staff bending close, their sleeves brushing mine, food delivered, everyone is happy, and I am surrounded.

If they could ignore me, it would be better. Let them talk to each other, let them not see me. Then at least I could eat or maybe watch them and have the time pass. But they include me, they don't want to leave me out and I listen to everything said for when they want to bring me back in. They ask questions and I answer, concentrating to work out when they are talking to me.

Even going to the bathroom is torture. I know the blessed cubicle awaits, the momentary stillness of a place with only me in it. Getting there is another matter.

Leaving the table, feeling the need to make some explanation of leaving the table, negotiating the walkways and acknowledging people on my way past. Through the doors, wondering where the toilets are, wondering if they will be signposted, if the staff will be there to tell me, if they will be full or if I can sneak into a cubicle and rest until I don't feel like crying.

The few minutes I can afford in solitude are worth the journey back to the table, almost worth having to sit down again, sometimes enough to help me through the rest. The quiet of the bathroom is what reminds me that, once home, I can have that quiet with no time limit.

Lifetimes later, the wedding is over. The panic thrumming its fingers on the edges of my eyes has dissipated. I can go home, I can go home!

And I swear:

I am never feeling this again.

When life seems unreal

Anxiety and Aspergers, the big double-act. Aspergers compelled to take centre stage, Anxiety in the back, making sure music is cued, the lights are right, trapdoor set for the comedy reprise. Just as important but rarely recognised, anxiety is the other side of the Aspergers conundrum.

Does a person with Aspergers 'act out' because of anxiety? Would they be able to cope better if they weren't anxious? Yes to at least one of those. I challenge anyone to cope better *with* anxiety than *without* it! What I take issue with is the inherent subtext, that if you take away anxiety, you mute Aspergers.

It's like saying the person will no longer have Aspergers if they aren't anxious – it doesn't make sense and has the convenient, offensive implication that someone who stifles their anxiety can also stifle their disability.

The truth, the hard reality, is that anxiety is a deeply-entrenched part of Aspergers for many people. The background music to the main event, without which you may have less drama, but you still have an aspie. Yet controlling anxiety is the holy grail in many families, with hope set firmly on making life easier for the loved one with Aspergers by maintaining calm.

The assumption is that an aspie without anxiety upgrades their chances of being a fully-paid cast member instead of a walk-on or understudy.

Sometimes being on the spectrum is like living half-in and half-out of the real world: surrounded by unreal people with strange, glimpsed motivations, left to figure out the plot at the same time as being a part of it.

Like a TV town by the sea, life seems populated by stereotypical characters who have their roles to play and know them off by heart. I have a role too, but I don't ever seem to quite learn the lines or know which door to leave by and when to come in on cue. Rather like the innocent niece or nephew on Murder She Wrote, sooner or later I find myself under suspicion, hoping for a kindly Aunt Jess to bail me out and explain it all away.

It's not just the people who seem unreal: colours boost or fade, impressions of a familiar room change as the light is adjusted behind the scenes and not by any switch I can reach. Shadows disappear in a harsh light or gather in new places - how did I never notice before that dark gap between the cupboard and the door?

The light caught in the window, reflecting through this morning's rain, takes on a quality reserved for mystical waking moments, as if I never saw rain before.

I know people are real, I will have seen the gap before, I can look at rain and see water. Yet there is a kind of side-effect, an overspill from using too much energy to deal with the real, uncompromising world around me.

If you look at something hard enough you start to see it differently, and so it is with people. If you watch to see what they do, to see what *you* should do, to see how they seem to feel and if it relates to you, they become more than people. They become *A Study in People*, and when you study something you're likely to get good at it.

Except that people are all different. You study **one**, you hope to know them **all**. It turns out you know **one**, and then often get it wrong. The studious act of controlling anxiety by understanding people is undone - and amplified - by the individuality of others.

Studying also has the ironic effect of separating you from people at the same time as involving you with them. Close enough to study, you might forget to interact: *being* human, being yourself, is secondary to *understanding* human.

It turns out that studying yourself is much more reliable. Other people change and are unpredictable, whereas you know exactly how unpredictable you are and might see it coming. Knowing yourself first and others second means you can plan ahead too – a bonus level in controlling anxiety.

For instance, if the other person turns out to be hard to handle, rather than worrying about why, and possibly blaming yourself, you can focus on your own reactions, reasons, motivations.

This kind of self-care is one major tool in dealing with anxiety. If you can't understand or handle other people, that is an anxiety alarm ready to go off. If you know what you will do if a situation becomes difficult, you have A Plan. Having a plan means you have an exit, and exits are brilliant.

Unpredictably, some people turn out to be brilliant too, and kind. These ones encourage you to focus on being yourself, they divert the lens away from working out what everyone else is doing. By being yourself, you find out who likes you as you are, and finding someone who encourages that behaviour *before they even know you* properly, can be life-changing.

As for the unreal moments, I've come to accept those too. Acting is second-nature to many aspies, why shouldn't the world be a little magical and unreal too?

And that dark gap between the cupboard and the door? Life always has those, it's part of the scenery.

Hypervigilance!

Being hypervigilant sounds like a super-power.

Instead of waiting to see how someone reacts *after* you have acted or spoken, study them *super-fast* before making your next move. Almost psychic, this gives you clues on what to do or say, and vital extra time to rein in planned eccentric actions/noises/information in your response.

(Notice how I say 'planned'. Nothing stops unplanned eccentric responses, this is why some dear people love us).

Conversations or interactions can only be made better by hyper-vigilance. Watch, watch, watch-deeper, watch-better, work 'em out: make them squirm under your laser stare, make them feel like the surface of the sun sears down on them. Make them yours.

Yes, and then? Then, after all that god-mode watching I have a good idea of how the other person is feeling and how they are reacting to whatever I have *already said and done*. But what if I haven't done anything yet? What if their reaction is at odds with my part in the interaction?

It's all very well studying my target but what use is it if I know *how* they feel but have no idea *why* they feel it?

Suddenly I am in the too familiar territory of Confusion. I said *this,* and they frowned - but I don't know why they frowned because *this* was a good thing and mild, yet they are frowning. I try again, building on the previous *this* with more goodness and mildness. Nope, it's worse, they're frowning more! What the heck?!

There's a point at which hyper-vigilance disintegrates, blowing away in the defeat of Confusion, leaving me with the certainty that no matter what I try to do, it will end up wrong. Confusion is kryptonite to hypervigilance.

No, I can't let it end! Looking back at the frowning person I try once more, try again to bring the good *this*-ness I hoped for before. Right, is that better?

Staring, waiting, mini-moments slipping by as I focus on their frown lines and that weird way people have of not being able to hold my gaze after all the times they tell me off for avoiding eye contact.

The conversation ends, the frown lifts long enough for the other to leave, making vague comments about having something to do. My great subject of *this*, my perfect *this*, lies ignored at my feet. Anger steps in.

'Why don't you want to talk about *this*?' I ask, harshly, hurt and confused.

The other person turns, another frown replacing the first, this one just as familiar - disbelief.

'I wanted to tell you about my problem!' they spit out, exasperated.

I shrug helplessly - people! 'Why didn't you say then?'

'I tried!' they cry, waving their hands a bit like I do. 'I couldn't get a word in edgeways once you started talking about *this*!'

They start to walk away, pausing only to call back, 'And anyway, you won't stop staring at me! It's off-putting!'

Hyper-vigilance is amazing when it comes to working out if people are happy, sad, angry, cheesed-off or fed up. Unfortunately, hyper-vigilance is rubbish at telling you *why* someone feels these things.

The superpower of being able to study people minutely sounds amazing, but like super heroes themselves, it's unusual for it to work in real life. I am left with scowls on both sides, and a hindsight-backside understanding of why.

This is why my chosen super-power would be mind-reading. It cuts through vigilance and I'd find out great stuff, as well as what they wanted to talk about. Either that or invisibility, then I could avoid Confusion and go for free ice cream instead (and the many other things we would all do if we were invisible).

We don't get to choose our super-powers, I am stuck with hypervigilance. Like any good hero, I train in my spare time and plot out how to win over those pesky villains and their tricks.

Sooner or later, this city and its secrets will be mine.

6: School days

An aspie at school

As a parent of an aspie school child, do you clench your jaw when the phone rings? Do you wonder each day if the teacher will call you in at home-time? When it is party time, are you worrying over whether your child will be invited? Or, worse still, inviting the whole class to your child's birthday but not knowing who will come?

Why does your spectrum child suffer anxiety through their school years when any child who attends somewhere for this length of time should be used to it by now?

Maybe the teacher is right, and your child is fine once you leave; maybe Aunty Joan is right, and you fuss too much? Maybe Mum is right, and your child is picking up on your anxiety? Or maybe *you* are right, and your child is suffering every time they go to school?

School can be familiar and terrifying at the same time. Believe me, it is possible to do something numerous times and still feel sick to your stomach at the thought of having to do it again. Just because a situation is familiar does not mean it is friendly, or safe.

I know school is relatively safe, but properly safe? Teachers are there to help and there are policies in place to stop bullying. There are rules and lumps and bumps of education. I know children go in every day and come out improved at the end of it.

I also know what it's like to go to school every day, and yet the days don't run into each other or tumble quickly, they exist separately, each one replaced by another and another.

This day I go to the classroom and it's okay; this day I go in and as I reach the classroom, I get shouted at. The next day I go in and I expect to be shouted at again. If it doesn't happen, I expect it to happen the next day. When it doesn't happen the next day, I wait to see how long it will be before it happens again because the awful truth of school is that events repeat.

I go in to school and to the classroom and there is more than one shout, or no shouts, or I get shoved, or that girl who hates me looks and makes faces. The teacher brushes past me and doesn't notice any of it; she smiles at the whole class and doesn't see me, and I realise how alone I am even though the room is packed. And I am too far from the door.

I wait for breaks with a dread I know other children do not feel: playtime is fun! Children play and laugh and run and meet their friends and everything is lovely.

Sometimes I play a game and don't know the rules. I make them up and I'm not asked to play again. If I know where to run and when to run, I still get it wrong because games are fluid.

Lunchtime comes and the packed lunch I bring makes me homesick because it was made at home on the counter in our kitchen. Homesickness fills me to the top, bunching up my stomach, making me nibble at the sandwich I wanted so badly minutes ago.

Then someone steals my sandwich or makes fun of it and they are attacking my home and what I love, and I don't feel safe again. I don't want to eat with them anymore. How do other people eat with all this going on? How do they learn the trick of not caring?

Later, safe at home, I try to explain, and I get a casual comment, like, 'They don't mean it, it's just the way people talk, maybe they want to be your friend?'

I remember the way they looked at me as they made fun and I know, even if I couldn't explain it, that they don't want to be my friend.

Some days, no matter how hard school was or how much I want to go home, I come out of the doors slowly, as if I can't be bothered to leave at all. There is a weariness to going somewhere each day.

It feels like I don't leave, even once I am safely home. And home doesn't feel truly safe when you know you must leave it again and go back to school.

The next day, leaving by the open gate, children rushing in like a glittering school of fish, I turn to check I if I can rush back out. Held by a need to be where I am supposed to be, I turn back in and join the school, swept through the doors and into the narrow halls.

Jess needs to try harder

Jess leaves her nice, warm bed and watches TV while she has her breakfast. The TV is just for fun, you know? But watching it makes her feel safe and comforted, the routine of her programmes enclosing her in the soft, strong, matchless security of home. She couldn't put it this way, she just likes her programmes.

Getting ready for school is a chore. She needs to be ready in time to leave, must start remembering things for herself, the way good children remember. She has to know where her bag is (here it is) and her shoes (under the bed) and keep her hair nice (we just brushed it!) and put her lunch in her bag (you almost forgot again!) and remember to give Miss the letter for the school trip (it's in your book bag).

Then once all this is done and in the right amount of time, home is left behind for another day.

Jess sees the other children going to school, some of them with parents, some striding out on their own, defiant and independent. Jess doesn't know they look this way, she only knows they walk on their own, crossing roads her mum makes her stand next to for ages in case a car is coming.

All the while, the air cuts through her school jacket, reminding her she isn't at home, in the warm. The sight of the other children makes her think of being at school all day with these strangers who run about and shout at each other and are a part of a great, big, little world where Jess is meant to belong.

At the school gate, Jess spots Kyle and looks away quickly. Kyle likes to tease her and dance about, rushing at her as if he will knock her right over, then missing at the last moment. Jess sees his mother grabbing him by the shoulder, spinning him to face her. It looks like he's already in trouble.

Kyle turns away from his mother and sees Jess watching. For a moment that exists outside of their school day, Jess sees the way his eyes look and then he pulls a face at being watched and turns away again.

The school door, full of people going in, crowded with parents leaving with happy faces. Jess's turn to go through and say goodbye and act like this is where she wants to be when the real Jess is still at home, in the warm, with no one pushing and jostling and no one shouting too loud and filling up all the space around her that she wishes was empty and quiet.

Only seconds later and she is alone in the classroom, though it is full. The teacher is making everyone calm down and Jess turns to the front and waits to see what she should do. She will be good all day and ask when she needs to do something and keep silent when she needs to know something.

Later, when Kyle has run past her a few times there will be another moment where, without knowing exactly why, Jess leans over and gives him her spare pencil because he has broken his own. And he'll twitch his nose at her in that way he does when he's making fun of the teacher, then laugh and nibble at the pencil she gave him.

Somewhere in the confused, inexplicable day of school the quiet, get-along girl will start to understand the loud, push-away boy, even if she couldn't explain to you what it is she knows about him. And the boy will look again at the silent girl who never asks for help and wonder if it really is because she knows all the answers or if she is lost too.

Many hours go by and Jess goes home again, relieved all the way through to leave school. A little rest (a full evening), a little sleep (a night full of dreams) and seconds later (the morning), then she will be back at school to do it all again and somehow *still*, even though this happens, her teacher will say,

'Jess needs to do better, we know she can. If only she would take part in lessons. Yes, of course she has friends! She's always in a group, doing something. No, we have no bullying at *this* school, we have a very clear policy.'

'Jess needs to try harder.'

Jess knows this is the face you make

Jess knows this is the face you make when you learn to read.

These are the eyes the teacher sees,

looking sideways to mimic reading.

This mouth, ready always to betray her,

opens and whispers a sound that could be a consonant.

All the time stalling, stalling, stalling,

in a sharp, 6-year-old hope

that the word will magically clear

by the time the sound reaches the air.

Jess knows this is the face you make when you learn to read, a little mouth, ready to open

and say the right word,

the eyes staring

at a blank-black-lettered page.

Her forehead most of all is what she shapes,

just the right force behind her frown

to make it seem she almost knows,

is on the very edge of knowing,

walks along the cliff-side,

ready at any nearby second to tumble

into a valley of knowing

where everyone else found their way by the easy path.

Jess sits after the teacher goes

and stares so hard at the old reading book

her head feels full of the girl on the cover

with her bucket full of gold.

Jess knows this girl doesn't need words,

she has her bucket of gold and her fairy-tale world.

Jess traces the picture with her finger and smiles

7: Communication

In celebration of oversharing

Oversharing is one of life's fundamental shortcuts: why spend weeks, months, years getting to know someone when you can find out most of it in the first half an hour? You don't have half an hour? You'd be surprised (and pleased) to discover how much fits into a few minutes.

It's not confined to Aspergers but oversharing is definitely a spectrum super-skill. It's the effervescent love-child of brutal honesty and naïve small talk. Springing up when there is a need or desire to be social, it exists mostly in aspies who have worked hard at holding conversations with others.

If you've needed to learn how to talk to people the 'right' way, the difference between normal social chatter and deeper, more revealing words becomes blurred. If I'm asked what I like doing, I tell people, and the answer might spread from a one-word answer to sentences of explanation.

As well as accounting for short, failed conversations, this spreading effect also creates unexpected friendships.

Giving more of an answer than is expected, means the other person sees a fuller version of you, and quickly. If they stick around after that, there's a better chance of them staying for more than one, over-full conversation.

It's not that I plan to share everything; once the words start it's hard to stop.

If the conversation is about the weather then I talk about the weather: rain, snow, what was predicted, what we got - global warming, natural disasters; eventually Space.

If it is about puppies, it becomes kittens, guinea pigs, foxes, mongoose, snakes – puppy farming, pedigrees, border collies, poop. The narrative flow is a hillside stream, staying connected but going where it likes.

An innocent conversation about the other person's house becomes a slow-reveal about my own house; and by slow, I mean I take a few sentences to describe my living situation instead of one.

Startled by oversharing, the other person will either tidy up the conversation and leave, try to change the subject (**ha**!) or be interested/confused into revealing more about themselves, or ask a question (bless them).

The lid is off then, I can overshare as much as I like. *They* asked a question, they want to know! And with this confidence, I reply in full detail.

There is sometimes a part of me looking on which wonders if this is the right thing to do, but mostly this part doesn't stir until it's over.

I am glad to share, with lacklustre success at holding back anything personal. Someone who shows a vague interest in my life will end up knowing more than they expected. Unfortunately, this is where I leave myself open to unscrupulous people who would rather use what they know than make a friend.

The after-thoughts, or regret, are a good time to consider if this person is okay, if I want them to know more – even if it's too late to hold back. The conversation itself might lay me open to bad people, but then I hope instinct and life experience kick in afterwards and alert me to anything off, or wrong. Tricky, a balancing act, but still...

The times I have left somewhere and realised, even as I

walked away, that I overshared again. Again, again. Mostly I shrug it off - there are too many 'agains' to worry about.

Sometimes I wince all the way home, replaying what I shared, how I said it, seeing in my mind's eye the truth of their expression which I glossed with enthusiasm the first time around.

A lot depends on the nature of the person who found themselves in the flow of that hillside stream: did they hop from stone to stone to get across or paddle in it, trying to get used to the currents?

Why am I celebrating oversharing? Does it not seem bad to lay your life open to a passing stranger or an acquaintance who asks a vaguely relevant question?

Categorically, it is worth celebrating. Blurt it out, readers, let it free. For every wince, every 'again' where you showed yourself to be **different** - there are times when the other person ends the conversation with a smile.

If the end goal was to make friends each time, that doesn't happen. If what you wish for is meaningful social interaction, a smile is a good start.

They may know more about me but often I come away knowing more about them too. There are people out there in this cynical world who react well to oversharing.

By being too open and overly honest, you give others the chance to repay the compliment. A fresh breeze springs up, the air clears, the sun is bright (for the time of year), and there is honesty between you.

Truth, like oversharing, can be catching. And the next time you meet, you might talk about more than the weather.

Logic vs sensibility

Logic dictates…sensibility feels.

Logic feels like being free: I love to explain, to describe, to show how it is, to discuss with another person. Sensibility would tell me when to start speaking or when to shut up.

Imagine: my friend always packs their shopping bags the wrong way. One day I explain the right way. I take care to be subtle and calm, positive that no feelings were hurt. Except then my friend is snappy about it and makes out they know how to pack their bags.

(obviously they *don't* know, or I wouldn't have had to tell them)

((but *now* they know))

I'm thinking that feelings were hurt because those bags had been packed wrong all this time, or because my friend can't take good advice when it's given? Or, um, maybe they loved that old way of packing bags? I don't know, I have no idea, but I realise that feelings were hurt despite my best efforts to be helpful.

Logic kicks me when it comes to other people. Logically, my friend should want to know how to pack their bags and should definitely want to know if they have been doing it wrong. Why wouldn't they want to know? That doesn't make sense.

Its illogical not to care about squashed bread or cracked eggs. Why would she put meat in with the fruit? Doesn't she understand cross-contamination? (She does now). And what is she thinking, putting the magazine in with the apples? Is she 5?

When I have it in front of me I can see exactly how I come across and I would be annoyed too. Even then, I assume it's the kind of anger that happens when someone realises they were doing it wrong, that I irritated them by pointing it out.

Until the next time we go shopping, and bread is flailing under tins, strawberries are squeezed against a squidgy packet of mince and the magazine is *rolled* into the space next to the apples.

My words not only fell on deaf ears, I now must fight the urge to repeat myself, or never go shopping with them again.

Later, much later, usually after consulting with someone else, I discover my friend was upset because I was critical of them in a public place, ie the checkout, and wouldn't take their hint to keep it down. Also, as they didn't seem to be listening, I raised my voice and did that thing with my glasses.

(I think that last part must be subjective, I can't be like that really).

Once this is explained, sensibility surfaces long enough for the familiar sinking feeling but not long enough to make any real difference. My need to explain the logical and reveal the illogical is too groovy to resist.

It is great, though. Here is this piece of information you may not know! I found it for you. I will help you to understand. I will expound the virtues of this information, wherever we are and for as long it takes.

It does not matter if you have heard it before – you must

need to hear it again, if I have noticed you doing something contrary to the information. Therefore, be still, there is no stopping me: my logic will prevail against your outdated sensibilities.

The next time we go shopping together - and it may be a long time - I will remember not to tell you how to pack your bags and I may even notice your nervous glances as you wait for me to say something. I will also notice the meat is now separate from the other food but that you still like squashed bread.

My inspirational presentation of the real-life effects of cross-contamination is vivid enough to stick with anyone.

You're welcome.

I need to tell you that you're wrong

If you're wrong, I do need to tell you. Especially if I have proof you're wrong. I'm sure you'll appreciate me whipping out my phone to show you the text you sent me on March 15th at 17.02, which stated that...

And this text shows that I am right, which means you are wrong and were also wrong the last time you mentioned it when you tried to tell me I was mixed up.

At this point it becomes apparent that you don't appreciate me telling you because you lose your temper and/or walk off. Leaving me holding the phone, re-reading the message with a confused nod, wondering why this didn't turn out better.

Yes, I do realise people take badly to criticism – I hate it too! I just can't figure out why they also take badly to the truth, especially when it is given to them matter-of-factly and with proof.

If I was wrong, as I so often am, someone offering me proof would (*inflame me, cause a meltdown, tears, make me feel bad*) be extremely useful because I like to have the facts. Why don't you want the facts?

It does feel unfair. As an aspie who is wrong *a lot*, I am used to people explaining how things are, or to them being confused when I act on my information – which was wrong – and come up against their reality.

This is why it becomes important to prove I am right on those occasions when I actually am right. To be told then, too, I am wrong, reverts me to a justice-filled child who knows it was her turn on the paint and Barry pushed in and the teacher believed him when he said it was his turn, meaning I have to wait another week!

Without proof, I am still this child; I know I am right and want you to believe me. My evidence is circumstantial to you but concrete to me. The frustration of not being believed is bitter.

And *with* proof? Well then, ho-ho! wait right there while I get it! Proof, I love it! Right in front of my eyes, right in front of *your* eyes, right there to show anybody who will listen (I am insufferable), proof that this time I am right.

It does make me sound like I gloat over the proof, and I

believe it comes across that way too. It's not true, though. What looks like gloating, and sounds like it, is actually triumph, barely ever achieved and savoured like the still-beating heart of my enemy.

Triumphantly presenting the proof means we can both know the truth; beautiful, factual truth which doesn't rely on my memory or perspective to make it real. Perhaps I do sound smug, if smugness is triumph mixed with a deep sense of relief that, this time, I can make it right.

To see you walking off after all that is mystifying. For heaven's sake, I have proof! and now we can decide on what to do next with full possession of the facts. Just when we were getting somewhere, you march off to aggressively wash pots or vehemently mop the floor you only did this morning. None of that makes sense, you know.

Which is why I follow you, still holding the phone. There is no escape from the truth. I think maybe you didn't realise? I feel anxious, as you have a face of thunder and keep splashing me with dirty water by accident. But I'm not put off...

Looking back, much later, sometimes years later, I see how annoying I must have been. I'm sorry if I was annoying and didn't understand you weren't really wanting to do the dishes or the floor. We were in the middle of a conversation and it was important to me to make sure it was right, what we were saying.

I can understand you felt angry and criticised, because you told me you felt this way. It might take me a while to make the link between your feelings and anything I said, though. Maybe if I had only read from the phone instead of trying to hold it up to your face? I thought you didn't realise what I was reading, you see, and might want to read it yourself.

I can't understand why you didn't tell me how you felt at the time. I would appreciate the feeling of being overwhelmed by emotions because I get that a lot myself. It wouldn't have stopped me showing you the phone, but it might have stopped me following you to the kitchen afterwards.

Years later, with all these understandings finally in place, and my empathy sitting on the table like a polished cup, I can still clearly remember the details of my rightness. And the angry thumping of the mop against the kitchen table legs, the slamming of the dishes onto the drainer and the sideways look on your face which saw that I was there, again, and in the wrong.

Being socially awkward

I have it down to a fine art, being socially awkward.

I cover it with the role of Friendly Person, changing my face, my voice, even what I might talk about. I am friendly, but find it hard to show it sometimes, so playing the role of 'friendly' makes up for my stone-faced, monotonous reaction when I'm not paying attention.

This is a way of getting by, especially if *small talk* is involved.

I am a short-lived Queen of Small Talk. My favourite is the weather because I like talking about the weather. I'm not as good at slotting in other subjects for tiny chats, it's the weather or whatever you bring up.

Chitter-chatter when I am feeling on top of things is fine, I can do it. The pretence lasts long enough for me to be a Friendly Person. And then...

The times when the Friendly role won't fit, like waking up and being two clothes-sizes bigger overnight. I get up, do what I always do, and it won't fit. The small talk that worked yesterday doesn't work today.

The words I normally use, sentences well-worked and easy, come out wrong, *off*. I can hear them: the dread tone, the muffled feeling of not having it quite right, like I'm almost proficient in a foreign language. Like an old war movie, I am the spy who suddenly says 'Green-witch' instead of Greenwich. (Grennich is the way it is pronounced).

My smile, it doesn't work either. I can tell my face is doing something else, though I have no idea what. I stop myself patting it, to see what it feels like. Physically, I feel like my face is stiff. I pull faces to loosen the muscles and try smiling again – terrifying.

Oh! for the ability to be socially adept for a couple of minutes at a time! But no, it isn't that easy. Socially awkward days will not be hidden, mistakes happen. And it's not only small talk that suffers.

Easy conversations are suddenly hard. My phrases fall apart, the conversation wavers in a heat haze. I am in the middle of it, trying to make it stay in one place, watching the other person to see if they notice I'm doing it wrong. (I do recognise this behaviour makes me no less awkward).

Invariably, I say something kind of stupid - not fully stupid, just stupid enough. And then try to cover it up, which of course is putting make up on a pig.

Good grief, why do I bother?!

Well, mainly because I'm forced to talk a lot for work and it's best to come across as friendly when you are tutoring other people's children. Usually it's fine and social and I don't mind. Then on the days I do mind and it isn't social, it's awkward because *I* am awkward. The whole thing becomes *awkward*.

One lucky aspect is that tuition means seeing various people in small-ish time slots: if I show myself up, it's over quite quickly and I move on to the next person - and do it all again. Though I might cringe each time, each person only suffers it the once.

The next time I see them I am hopefully back to 'normal', with no weird, half-born smile and no stupid comments either. Back to desperately covering up the fact I am totally, irredeemably socially awkward.

Bliss for those times when I meet someone worse than myself! The empathy is palpable, as is my relief that I don't have to worry over odd comments on the weather labelled with wrong smiles.

Like-minds isn't just about being able to talk about the same things; sometimes it's listening to someone else make a hash of it and knowing exactly how they feel.

The only fix I have found for being socially awkward is to stop caring, as much as possible. I am human, contrary to how it appears when I fail at smiling: I do care if our social interaction goes wrong. I crawl into my car, thud the wheel, make an animalistic noise into the waiting air and drive away to do it all again.

Knowing it will be done again is the key to not caring about awkwardness. It's exhausting to care about each mistake. Why waste energy when I'm doing my best?

Why chastise myself when I have come out today and managed work, doing what I need to on a day when I would rather be at home?

I made it, I am here. If it is the right day for a wrong smile, look away or show me how it's done.

8: Empathy

Showing empathy

Imagine being on the outside of a shop with a big, bold window decal advertising what looks like a giant salad.

From the outside looking in, you see nothing of the shop. You have no idea if the salad is giant-sized or has sold out. You must trust that something is going on behind the decal besides giant salad. The salad advert is a specific image on the outside of the shop, how ridiculous would it be to expect the inside of the shop to be wall-to-wall giant salad?

Inside the shop, looking out, we discover it's a 2-way decal and the outside world is visible. Like an enormous pair of multi-coloured decorated sunglasses, the shop windows are covered in the giant salad advert.

From this side, I can see through green lettuce to the green road and shades of green cars, see the faces of passers-by reddened by radish, paled by sliced onion, split-second picklings as they walk by the cucumber.

The world outside is not the giant salad, though that's what I look through from inside the shop. I can see the world, I know it's inches away. The world is real, so is the shop and the decal in the middle.

This colourful barrier, designed to show the outside world what the shop needs it to see, is how I feel empathy is presented by people on the autistic spectrum. We are not empathy-free zones – far from it.

There is the world, a step or two away. Inside the shop. it's busy, there's plenty going on and the shelves are stocked. My current reaction is 'giant salad', a primary image displayed to the outside world.

A sad event - giant salad. Terrible news - giant salad. Happy, joyous news – salad. New baby – hiding behind the salad.

Just because all you see from the outside is salad, doesn't mean that's all there is in the shop. For Pete's sake, it's a *shop*...why would there only be salad? Even a greengrocer's stocks more than salad!

The supposed real world, the one outside the shop, is definitely there, though it feels less real when ensconced inside the warm, familiar shop. People allowed in here are also familiar, this is an establishment very particular about its clientele.

The giant salad in the window has a dual purpose: I can see out without others seeing in, and it shows the outside world only what I want it to see.

By hiding my feelings, I hide the whole inside of the shop. It is hard to let people look in without them seeing everything – you cannot stop people seeing what is visible, either you leave your windows free or filter what is on view.

As it's complicated to keep changing what people see, it might be that bigger, more emotional news is met with a similar reaction. I might (subconsciously) choose a certain reaction for *insert emotional event*. If I'm not showing appropriate gladness/sadness at your news, it could be this is my reaction to glad/sad news, make the best of it.

Inside, I may be thinking, *Wow, Stacey and Alan are having a baby at last, after all their years of trying. They must be incredibly happy, I'm happy for them too.*

If I allow myself to think about what Stacey and Alan have gone through to get their baby, I am in danger of being consumed by their suffering, their reactions to each failed attempt. I can visualise their tears so strongly, I start crying myself.

The great news that they are finally becoming parents is too much. If I feel that too, what can I do? I will be lost in their kaleidoscope of emotions; I won't be able to process the kaleidoscope, only feel it and see it.

Letting all of it in, the outer me will be a trembling mess, not displaying the depth of my emotion. I am more likely to look as if I am about to pass out or throw up. Not the reaction Stacey and Alan were hoping for.

Instead, I give them the standard glad/sad reaction, holding my empathy on the inside for fear of becoming them, in that moment. I avoid being drenched in empathy, they avoid an inappropriate reaction. Unfortunately, they might also avoid a great reaction and leave thinking nothing in this world touches me.

I would almost rather give in and be more than is expected, than be blank-faced, impassive, saying words that sound untrue because it is my steady, monotonous voice speaking them. Would they cope any better with an over-reaction, though? People might avoid telling me anything.

Don't set her off, you know what she's like.

She must be putting it on, nobody's really like that.

In my shop, faces are shaded by the decal, words are muffled by the windows. I might suspect what you say and know you talk about what goes on in here, this place you cannot access. I know part of the intrigue is my inaccessibility. Curiosity makes others come close and stare at the decal, as if I cannot see them do it.

It was placed there with the express purpose of protecting what I have inside and showing you what I think you need to see. I know the road is not green, and your face is not pickled: you know there must be more than giant salad inside my shop. Somewhere between these two lies the truth of what we have together.

If you stand close to the window and try to see in, you will only see the decal in detail. Be sure, if you do try, I am on the other side, looking out, closer than I might have been, almost touching the glass, studying you to see if I should open the door.

Selfish empathy

I have found it easier to empathise with a passing stranger than a loved one. What does that say about me? I'm assuming it says I am selfish.

It is possible to obsess on the idea of how someone not connected to me feels yet ignore the feelings of those closest to me. This strange double vision impacts on my place in the family, as well as my reaction to social situations.

So it is that an acquaintance and their problems might be on my mind to the point that I dream of them, I see their emotions, can imagine a path through their thoughts and feelings. In person I might say nothing to them and have no thought beyond trying to behave normally because to bring up their situation is beyond our friendship level. (I have been burnt too many times by imagining friendships where they didn't exist to risk it without caution).

Then to my loved ones: they're sad, in the depths of something great or awful, and what happens? I might worry about them but also still snap at them for leaving the milk out or forget that they are sad and become annoyed when they don't listen to my conversation. What is it all about?

How can it make sense to feel more for an acquaintance than a loved one?

It makes sense when you realise that to feel this worry *with* your loved ones, as well as *for* them, is to descend into palpable, unguarded empathy; to admit a weakness sharp enough to break the dam. Empathy dissolves barriers between us and I am left in a flood-rush of feelings and fears with nothing to hold them back.

Why should facing the flood stop me from being empathetic? Why would I care for myself first and my best beloved last? Why, if I daren't allow empathy, can I not even show sympathy?

Sympathy is a whole other issue because it's entirely possible to feel empathy and still not show sympathy: feeling and showing are two separate states. Feelings happen by themselves whereas *showing* sympathy takes effort, both to admit some feeling from yourself and the ability to communicate this, verbally or otherwise.

Add to this the issue of touch – people often expect physical contact if they know you well and you are expressing sympathy. How to make a lack of sympathy worse? Push someone off when they want a sympathetic hug or freeze as they come at you. They might know you don't 'do' hugs, but this isn't a normal situation, therefore **HUGS**.

Simplistically, avoiding a loved one's suffering is ignoring something and hoping it will go away. It doesn't often go away (though the loved one might, if we carry on), but hoping it can be avoided is easier than dealing with a torrid mix of emotions, people and awkward social skills.

Simpler still, logic loves fixes and aspies often try to solve problems by offering solutions. Fixes and solutions are comforting, they make problems manageable, they make them go away.

Someone who needs empathy does not always, or even often, want a solution. This is confusing. Why would someone not want a solution? There might not be one, perhaps nothing can be done; but if it can be done, why not try it? And if you haven't thought of the solution, why not listen to mine? Why is it not welcome?

Frankly, this one goes into the 'Other' folder. I want solutions, crave them. Other people don't want them, they crave empathy instead. Other people are not me, I understand that, even if I don't understand the need for comfort over solutions.

If my empathy shows, I want you to know I care. I'd rather not hug you to show I care, I will try not to recoil if you move in though. Hugs are not dangerous, I'll repeat it and hope the hug helps, and quickly.

If I offer solutions, please try not to reject me, it's extremely confusing. If I am overwhelmed by feelings, as you might be, a solution calms me and gives me focus. I don't understand what your focus is, or why you'd rather hold my hand than let me use my hand to write a plan.

Remember I care and will spend days and nights reliving what bothers you, imagining it from your point of view, feeling it as if we shared the same breath.

I might not do hugs or hand holding, but the distance

between us is filled with love for you.

Personal empathy

When I was eight years old, my grandfather became very ill and almost died. We were best friends who had adventures together; looking back, I believe Granda was on the spectrum. I wasn't allowed to visit him in hospital because he was too poorly. Once he was home, I was taken to visit.

I was afraid because his bed was in the front room and the old, grey man in the bed didn't look like my tall playmate and fellow adventurer. He was pale and weak but trying to be normal for me. Everyone told me he was a lot better and that I should try to cheer him up. For some reason, they trusted me alone with him.

I had the bright idea that guinea pigs would cheer him up – they always made me happy and he bought me my first piggies. So…I brought my guineas to see him and let them loose in his bed, sliding them in under the covers next to his enormous feet.

It livened things up, I can tell you. Poor Granda woke to the feel of fur on his ankles and the sight of lumps moving under the covers, coming up the bed towards him. I'm not sure how much it cheered him up, but it brought colour to his cheeks.

When I was twelve, he told me of the near-death experience he had when he almost died in the hospital (before coming home to my guinea pigs). He thought he was back in the coal mines and down a deep, narrow mine shaft. People above were letting giant rocks fall down the shaft - boom! boom! boom! - and each rock blocked out the light as it fell so that when he looked up, the light kept shutting out. This was when they were shocking his heart back to life, but in his mind, he thought they were burying him, and he woke with a deep sense of dread.

This later conversation, of rocks falling into mines, death and life thereafter, cast him as my fellow adventurer again, rather than a grandad who needed help. To admit his fear was not something he could do. By painting it as a supernatural and dreadful tale, I was fascinated and less afraid myself.

I didn't have the understanding to work out he was talking about being afraid or upset, I only knew his near-death experience took him back to times in the mines when he thought he would never see light again.

We were in the middle of an outdoor market at the time. He needed to rest, and I stayed with him while my grandmother and her friend inspected underclothes and the mysterious allure of new tea towels. In the sunshine, next to a green and black pillar meant for Victorian market stalls, an engrossed girl and her storyteller grandfather had a conversation that, from a distance, looked like any other.

We talked about a dread mine-shaft and the philosophy of death, but not how it made him feel. Neither of us thought about how it made *me* feel, to imagine losing my grandfather. We were both wrapped up in the story at the time.

For the rest of his life, when it came to illness, he expressed his physical ailments in exquisite detail and imagination but couldn't bring himself to say that he was afraid. You had to look for it in his voice, his words, the way he relied on stories from the mines to describe terrifying times.

And to him, what could be said? Emotions startled him, as if I was suddenly shouting. He didn't know what to do with me if I showed emotion, though he was emotional in his own way. My Grandma would raise her eyebrows at the pair of us and look at the fire to contain her amusement.

You see how a whole emotional relationship was built on not bringing out into the open feelings which ran close under the surface? How could I look at this man who was like a father to me, and see how he felt and know how I felt and yet have neither of us speak about it all the time we were together?

In the end, I realised this was how we dealt with our empathy.

He was old and in terrible health, but if we pretended this wasn't true (ignoring it so it might go away), then he wouldn't die.

He wouldn't die if we didn't express that he might die. He wouldn't die even when railing at his relatives for not visiting him when he might be lying dead for all they care. He wouldn't die if, somehow, he could get out of bed in the morning and put his best-grip hand on the walking frame.

If he could frame-it down to the pink roses by the gate and smell them, then he wasn't dying either. Sitting on the low wall by the rise in the pavement, that meant he wasn't dying. Watching his corner of the world go by meant he was not dead.

His adventures continued, down to the roses and just beyond: as long as he had them, he would not die. He could talk to us about the scent from the roses, the weather today, who he could see in the distance going to the shop, who saw him and waved, who came to talk to him, 'Jackie, lad!' to tell him the news.

Translate it, if you need to; in his last adventures he poked a thumb at every morning that wanted him dead and took it as a personal victory to prove that morning wrong. He didn't want our sympathy, he wanted the kind of empathy that would ask him about the roses, what so-and-so bought at the shop and revel in giving us gossip before we heard it ourselves. This was what he craved.

I stood, watching from my window, terrified he would fall.

My Grandma surreptitiously watched from the front room. I felt the eyes of our close neighbour upon him and sometimes she would wander out to do light gardening nearby where he was.

Inside, restored to his role as conqueror, he told us how he suspected Greta was waiting for him to fall, that she was nosier than ever. Refusing to see her empathy meant he could be normal with her.

When he died, I didn't wear black. I bought a dress of purple, pink and blue and strode into the funeral. I would not be going to his last goodbye wearing a dress the colour of rocks, or mine walls.

If I wore roses, he could not die.

9: Being yourself

How can I change?

Imagine being muddy from a long mountain hike.

My legs ache, I cannot wait to rip of my muddy boots, pull out the too-thick socks caked in drying, swamp-green water. My trousers changed colour too and I think they could stand up by themselves.

My face, glimpsed in the bathroom mirror, is covered in mud, a choice of shades. I can pick out the field mud from where I fell trying to get away from the cow.

What I wouldn't give to be in the bath right now. Blissful water soaking off the mud, easing my aches and pains.

What if I can't change?

I stand in a trapped loop at the mirror, examining my sad and dirty face staring back, right next to a steaming bath and the promise of relief and comfort.

Why do I not get in?

No one told me how to escape the loop. Like a trapped ghost doomed to repeat the same small seconds of life:

consider, decide, fail to move, repeat. Comfort waits behind me, out of sight.

Why can't I move?

Is it quantum physics and I am a multi-me, caught when we triggered some gazillion-to-one spatial loop?

The bath waits, frustratingly now at a perfect lukewarm temperature. Steam coats the walls, condensates down the mirror, down me. A thin rivulet of once-was-steam tracks through mud on my face, leaving a trail of clean.

Perhaps the answer is not in a perfect solution?

This revelation grips me hard enough to startle and I fall back towards the bath. Staggering, I reach the water and plunge in my arm.

Mud balloons off, rising like ash from a fire, spilling out over the substitute heaven of Water over Bath. I wonder.

It is against normal rules. What will it look like? How will it feel? Why would a person do this?

I climb into the bath fully clothed. This time, mud does not balloon, it blossoms, an instant of flowering which fills the bath completely. I wallow in a mud-flower.

What now?

Still dressed, not clean, mud spattered on the tiles around the bath, the floor, the taps, even the window.

Once begun, change gains momentum. I climb back out, rinse the bath, fill it again, repeat. In a loop of my own making, I am improving with each repetition.

We must all find solutions best fitted to our unique predicaments. Later, I consider what I did wrong, what I did right. Why I could not change.

Waiting, I wonder if a solution will present itself. And while I wait, I dream.

Anyone can build a house

Imagine I have a new job at the building site. I have some experience at building work, I've learned the rules and regulations and carefully read the job description. Determined to make a good impression, I walk in and wait to be told what to do.

Around me there are lots of other people working on the site. It's big and there are a bewildering variety of tasks going on. I start to worry I might not be up to the job, but I did study and learn all I could… I try to relax.

Then the boss gestures to the corner of the site and says,

'Build the house there.'

What? A whole house? By myself??

Seeing me panic, he rolls his eyes and adds,

'Anyone can build a house, you should know what to do.'

I stare at him, as if this extra knowledge might sprout up from him and fly over to me. It doesn't.

Exasperated, the boss turns and leaves me to it. He doesn't have time to waste and, as he said, anybody can build a house.

I go to the corner of the building site and look at the spot where my house is to be built. The ground is dusty, a few pebbles scattered about, a lost nail from a nearby development. Close to the boundary of my patch, someone else is halfway through with their house. A distance away, a gleaming row of houses is being admired by the person who built them single-handed, from scratch.

Is this how building is supposed to work? All by myself in a corner of the site with only my two hands and mysterious, innate knowledge to guide me? Perhaps I could ask for help?

Comparing myself to the others, I realise I am hopelessly out of my depth. Even if I ask for help, I would still have no real idea what I was doing. Shouldn't there be training for this? How come everyone else knows without being trained? Was there training and I missed it?

An instruction book would be good right now. The rules

and regulations I read to prepare me don't help with this, they only gave a broad outline of what I should and shouldn't do. They don't explain this specific situation; it is assumed I understand.

Anyone can build a house, if by anyone you mean any other person but me, and people like me.

This house has more chance of building itself, four walls rising with dignity from the lusty ground, reaching for the air as tiles fly in to populate the growing roof. Windows backwards jump like gymnasts into waiting sockets, each one clicking shut. The door takes a running jump and lands squarely where it should, polished and ready to lock.

This does not happen, leaving me to stand and study the dusty earth, safe in my hard hat and high-vis vest, which I wore because I read the rules.

Anyone can build a house. Can anyone help me?

Aspie mimic, aspie mime

There's a little girl at the end of her group of friends – she calls them friends but only one of them ever comes home with her for tea. She watches as the girl at the opposite end to her tells a story. The other girls lean in to hear as well as watch.

Our little girl leans in, watching, listening, vacuuming up the mannerisms of the other, taking in her tone of voice, tilt of her head, the way her eyes tell the story and wait for a reaction at the same time.

This other, polished girl has a flounce in her hair when she moves her head: our little girl gently moves her own head in a flounce, feeling her hair shift, noting what makes it happen.

The other girl tells the middle of the story, the part where she is almost at the point of adventure. Her audience is rapt. Our little girl stores the details of the story: at the same time, she breathes in the posture of the other, the foot placed heel-to-toe – how does she stand that way without falling? Our girl nudges her own heel to a toe and resolves to try it later.

Under this conscious study, our little girl is subconsciously noticing how others in the group react, their changes in posture, their laughter and the tones of their voices as they respond to the storyteller. This is what an audience looks like – a positive audience. Our little girl isn't sure about any of that, she doesn't have great memories of people watching her. Still, though, to be the centre of attention and know what to do with it!

Unbeknownst to her, our little girl stores away this memory of being comfortable in the spotlight, setting it next to contrasting memories of herself hating the spotlight. Even as she saves up vital details of how to be the storyteller, she creates a stored difference between herself and the girl telling the story: she takes on the mantle of being the opposite to this popular, sociable girl.

Multiply this event manifold, make it rush through a girl's life as she ages, bring us to the point when our little girl is starting yet another new job. By now she is in her late 20s, far too old to be in a playground group trying to take in the social basics.

Introduced to her co-workers, our girl follows their lead, is a quick study, even if she studies who to avoid and who to trust before she learns how to do the job. She is constantly learning, soaking it up now she is an adult.

In her new job she is surrounded by other adults, some older, some younger; understanding without being told that most of them know how to be the centre of attention, know how to stand heel-to-toe without falling. These years later, our girl has a two-fold storage process: useful information on how to behave and useful information on why she is not able.

Years pass, and the habit of learning never ends. It doesn't matter her age, or her life experience, each new social event is an opportunity to glean more knowledge of how she should be, of how others do it. She passes as one of them, she is one of them at times.

At the back of her mind is a box chock-full of comparisons, harsh and soft contrasts between herself and others. Here is the other side of her never-ending ability to learn and mimic people around her. A tumbled, spilling box of clothes not hers, forgotten faces, behaviours she cannot emulate: each one a piece of the greater assumption that she will never match up.

It is not simply self-esteem or lack of it: it is a carefully-learned perspective on how the world does not have quite the right space for someone who, metaphorically, cannot stand heel-to-toe without falling.

More years pass, the number of them individual to the girl. Here she is now, wondering what is wrong and why she cannot do what she always did – what she has studiously learned to do. Why now, after her triumphs?

Why should it be now, when she is more than fully grown, many years from the playground, that she feels herself grinding to a half and wanting to avoid everything she has struggled to gain in her life?

Why does she want to walk away? Dreaming of it more each day, as if she was dreaming of saving herself.

The box is hidden under a packed-in, shoved, wedged mountain of clothes which don't belong to her. Each face unlike her own has blended into the world itself, looking on. There is no path past the hidden box, no safe detour. Clambering over the top of it is unthinkable.

Why is it unthinkable? It is only a box, filled with clothes she collected. She put them there herself, didn't she?

She did, but mostly without thinking. She can pick out one or two familiar items, the rest are a mass of cloth she doesn't recognise.

It comes, the day when her mimicking cannot get her past the unseen box, and she doesn't have the resources to help her climb over it. By mimicking, she learned how to pass as similar to other people, if not the same. Being a mimic has served her well.

Now that she is called upon to find the initiative to climb over the mass of clothes, she looks into herself and finds only what she requires to behave like other people. It is herself who has this problem, not them.

Why does her looming mass of clothes feel intrinsically linked with dreams of freedom? Surely the unknown clothes trap her, rather than free her?

It comes, though it might be years. There is nothing to be done but climb over the clothes. Unbelievably, our girl managed to stuff even more in there while she was thinking about what life means. Now she has a vast pile to wade through or stumble over.

Standing silently, staring at what she must encounter next, our girl has nothing to say. At this point in life, mimicry fails her, and mime takes its place. She can only gesture her meaning, over-exaggerate what she does, mime in front of others and hope they understand because she cannot explain it to them.

She can still copy - miming is copying - but it is a ballooning, swelling version of the truth, writ large and seen clear from afar. Mimicking has installed in our girl an ability to present what she means to say without the capacity to explain her finer details.

She takes a step and her toe touches the cloth of the nearest garment. Why should she tumble, though? Is it promised?

Bending in her new, extravagant mime, she plucks at the cloth, pinches it tight, tosses it into the air and sees it fly against the light. She smiles.

It was almost a bird there, flying high, bright above her,

flapping as it fell, landing out of her path. She chooses another, does it again.

She doesn't smile at each one. Some clothes relive harsh comparisons minutely remembered. Pluck it, pinch it, toss it, hesitate over it when she must. They are all birds, some darker than others, taking flight above and landing away from her. She can see them where they land, see them clearly enough to identify them if she wants.

As she walks through the dwindling bundle of clothes, the ones she releases take less of her attention and she has to make a special effort to pick them out. She becomes less interested the more she clears a path.

The mime is silent, the message presented unspoken. Inside the mime, there is a person filled with words, letters closeted away in shining books our girl can hardly bear to touch. She touches them.

No mime needed now, she reads and devours her own words instead of the words of others. She studies her own behaviour, letting loose the behaviour of others.

She looks deep into her shining books and sees her

younger self smiling back, holding up childish hands to stretch the sky in her grandmother's garden.

The mimic and the mime are part of her, she can never leave them behind or free them like dark birds. What changed is how close this dancing, smiling girl is to the surface of her new life. It doesn't matter if she falls or cannot stand heel-to-toe – why did it seem this skill mattered above her other skills?

True to herself, our girl trips along the cleared path, full of illuminated words she wrote without knowing. Behind her, false birds lay scattered in the path, unrecognised.

10: Guides

How to give your aspie a quiet Christmas

How should you treat your aspie at Christmas time? Can enforced good cheer and sociability be avoided? And the more difficult question, what do you tell other people about your aspie and Christmas?

Please note

Avoid the obvious tactic of sticking a big sign outside your front door with your message of choice written on it.

People who want to visit you will ignore any sign, however big and obvious. It wouldn't matter if you painted, 'Feck off, Gladys' on it; Gladys would still knock at the door.

With that in mind...

1. **Tell people to stay away.**

Yes, stay away. Right away. Presents? Post them. Cards? Made for posting, damn it. Too late to post? We don't mind them late. Too stubborn to post things? Determined to deliver to your door? Deliver to the door then, don't expect it to open.

2. When your friends and family turn up at the door anyway.

Don't open the door, but if they peer at you through the glass, come out and wave them away like you would with pigeons.

3. When your friends and family think you haven't recognised them because you appear to be waving them away and not letting them in.

Hold up a pre-made sign with GET AWAY WITH YOU printed on it. Hold it close to the window as they scrunch their eyes up to read.

4. (Having decided you cannot be serious) **They knock on the window and ask if you are letting them in**.

At this point you may be tempted to fling open the door and ask if they remember the conversation you had only yesterday where you told them you were not having *any* visitors over the festive season because your aspie finds it too stressful.

Please resist this temptation.

Of course they remember the conversation, they just didn't think you meant *them*.

5. **Outside, a discussion takes place whereby your relatives decide how to deal with this latest madness from you.**

Take the opportunity to close the curtains while they are having the discussion. If you do not have curtains or your blinds are flimsy, lie down on the floor and pretend to be in a deep sleep.

6. **Your phone will now start ringing.**

It's strange how, having seen you only yesterday, during that conversation about keeping away, then having come today and been kept away by you, people who are wanting to visit will call you to see why you are not letting them in.

7. **If you have a toddler, or can borrow one, let them answer the phone.**

If you do not have access to this age group, please

make sure you have pre-recorded an answer phone message containing a small song about Not Today, Thank You. Singing answer phone messages are unnerving and get the job done.

8. **Be prepared, after all your efforts, for your aspie to ask why no one is visiting.**

The fact that your aspie hates these unexpected visits and detests opening presents in front of people means nothing at the moment of asking.

9. **Don't forget to spend at least half a day planning how next Christmas will be easier because (fill in the blank with whatever ruined it this year and why you're never doing *that* again).**

There is no explanation as to why we do this to ourselves every single year.

10. **If all else fails, utilise your giant GET AWAY WITH YOU sign.**

This counts as a Christmas craft and can be decorated with as much glitter as you like. It's also very therapeutic to fill in individual names on it, as you repel each visitor.

Above all else, do whatever it takes to have a Happy Christmas to suit you and your aspie.

For reference, here is the Not Today song, best sung in the style of Laurel and Hardy holding axes.

Not today, thank you

I want to be alone,

Not today, thank you,

Please don't even phone.

I want to have my Me Time

I want to lock the door,

And if you keep on phoning,

I'll not answer any mo-rrrre.

How to make friends with an aspie

Ask if they would like to be friends.

This high-risk strategy seems sensible, given what you know about making your intentions clear and not trying to hint at people on the spectrum. What could go wrong?

There may be an interlude reminiscent of Pinter where you listen to an inner monologue from your new friend as they explain they already have 2 friends, but 3 is still a prime number and if you only turn up when they ask or on the Thursdays when they are at home, it might be ok.

Please try not to be overwhelmed with the honest and random response given to this question.

Ask if they would like to be friends.

I have friends.

Short, brutal version of the previous reaction. Very likely followed up with an answer later, once you have accepted rejection and left.

If you are brave enough to proceed, carry on.

Ask if they would like to be friends.

Silence. Or pretence you never spoke. Looking away at a duck. Staring hard enough at your shoulder for you to stare too.

At some indeterminate point later, you will be given a short answer, by which time you need to decipher what they are answering because you are in the middle of buying duck feed.

Ask if they would like to be friends.

They say no and include reasons which become a valuable, revealing life-lesson, answering many questions about your past relationships.

Ask if they would like to be friends.

You are accepted into the fold of friendship with immediate effect and, depending on location, are dragged up to the collections room (be still, it's Star Trek), or stand for an hour in Tesco peering at pictures on a phone of what looks like a room full of tiny Vulcans.

Ask if they would like to be friends.

It will be explained how there are certain expectations to friendship, having been burned in the past.

There will be no turning up unannounced, for instance. Phone calls are a no, except if you have lost each other while out, and then only if all reasonable, non-verbal methods of communication have failed.

Ask if they would like to be friends.

Your other friends are not included in this deal. Maybe later, if you happen to mention one of them likes Star Trek.

Ask if they would like to be friends.

Your family is not part of the deal unless they have already been encountered and are satisfactorily uninterested in social interaction or offer good food (and don't ask questions while it is being eaten).

Ask if they would like to be friends.

Be prepared to explain why you want to be friends. What was it about the aspie that made you ask the question?

Please don't answer with generalisations or feelings. Scan your data banks: when did this idea occur to you and why?

If you don't have an answer, be prepared for a Spock-like eyebrow.

Ask if they would like to be friends.

You become friends.

Ask if they would like to be friends.

You're already friends.

By the same author

A Guide to Your Aspie

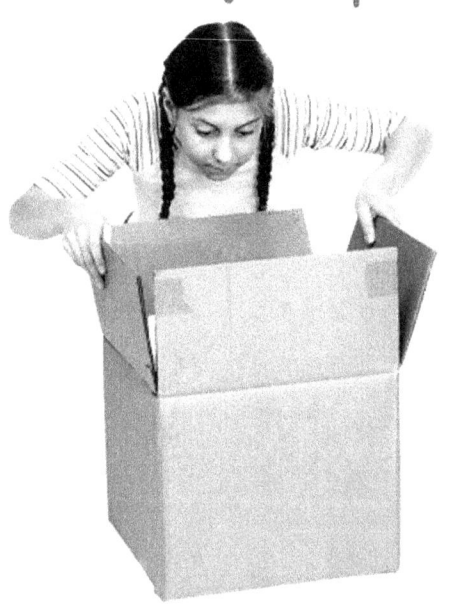

Amanda J Harrington

How to Talk to Your Aspie

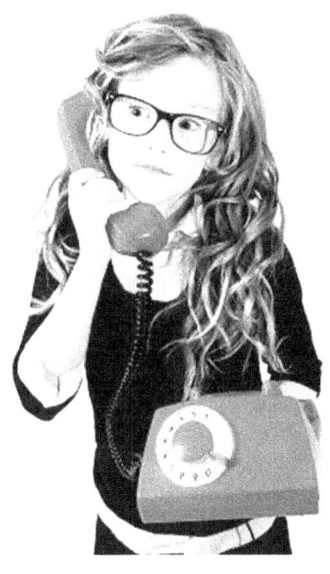

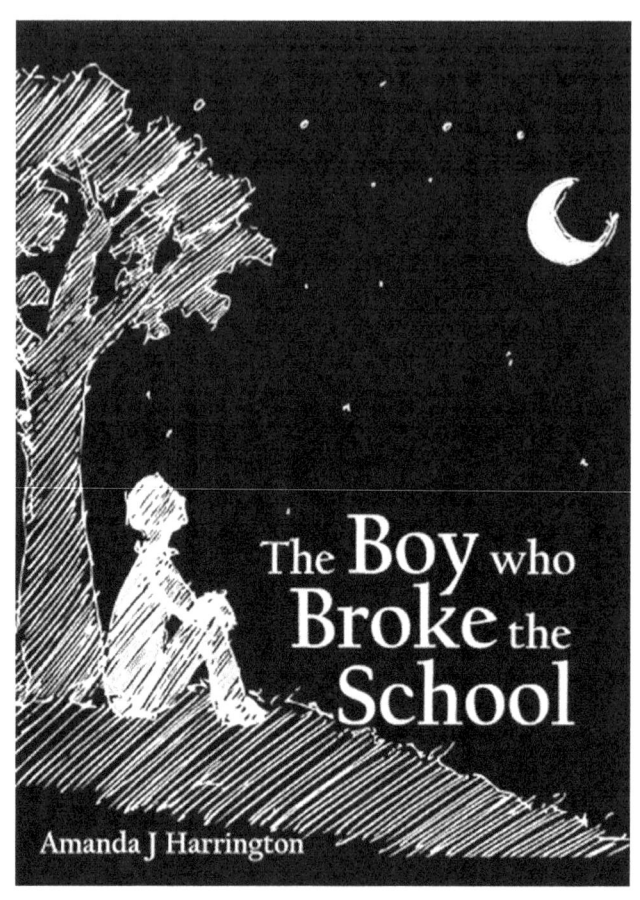

The Boy who Broke the School

Amanda J Harrington

A Crash Course in Creative Writing

Amanda J Harrington

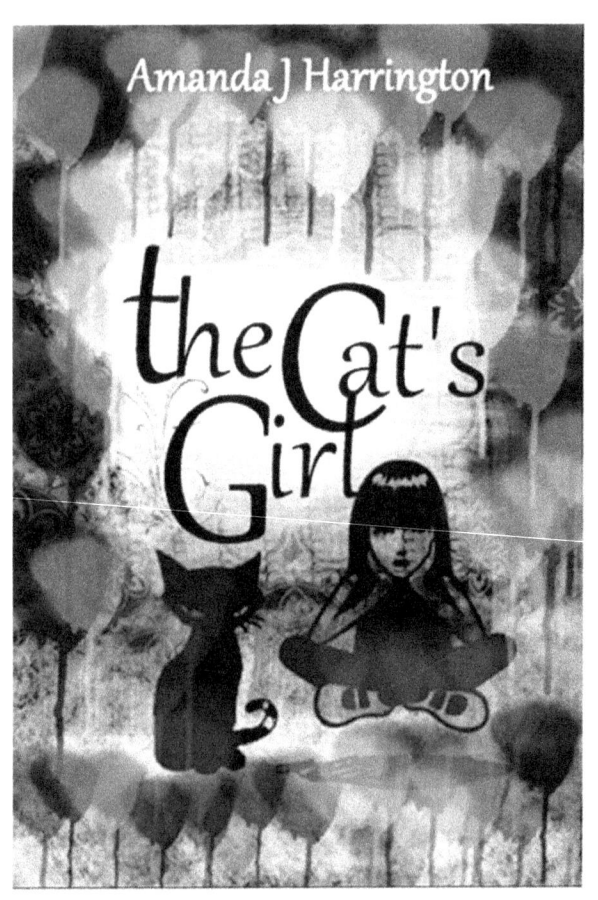